Surgical Challenges of the Foregut

Editor

SUSHANTH REDDY

SURGICAL CLINICS OF NORTH AMERICA

www.surgical.theclinics.com

Consulting Editor
RONALD F. MARTIN

June 2019 • Volume 99 • Number 3

ELSEVIER

1600 John F. Kennedy Boulevard • Suite 1800 • Philadelphia, Pennsylvania, 19103-2899

http://www.surgical.theclinics.com

SURGICAL CLINICS OF NORTH AMERICA Volume 99, Number 3
June 2019 ISSN 0039–6109, ISBN-13: 978-0-323-67805-6

Editor: John Vassallo, j.vassallo@elsevier.com
Developmental Editor: Meredith Madeira

Surgical Clinics of North America (ISSN 0039–6109) is published bimonthly by Elsevier Inc., 360 Park Avenue South, New York, NY 10010-1710. Months of publication are February, April, June, August, October, and December. Business and Editorial Offices: 1600 John F. Kennedy Blvd., Suite 1800, Philadelphia, PA 19103-2899. Periodicals postage paid at New York, NY and additional mailing offices. Subscription prices are $417.00 per year for US individuals, $845.00 per year for US institutions, $100.00 per year for US students and residents, $507.00 per year for Canadian individuals, $1071.00 per year for Canadian institutions, $536.00 for international individuals, $1071.00 per year for international institutions and $250.00 per year for Canadian and foreign students/residents. To receive student/resident rate, orders must be accompanied by name of affiliated institution, date of term, and the *signature* of program/residency coordinator on institution letterhead. Orders will be billed at individual rate until proof of status is received. Foreign air speed delivery is included in all *Clinics* subscription prices. All prices are subject to change without notice. POSTMASTER: Send address changes to *Surgical Clinics*, Elsevier Health Sciences Division, Subscription Customer Service, 3251 Riverport Lane, Maryland Heights, MO 63043. **Customer Service (orders, claims, online, change of address): Telephone: 1-800-654-2452 (U.S. and Canada); 314-447-8871 (outside U.S. and Canada). Fax: 314-447-8029. E-mail: journalscustomerservice-usa@elsevier.com (for print support); journalsonline support-usa@elsevier.com (for online support).**

Reprints. For copies of 100 or more, of articles in this publication, please contact the Commercial Reprints Department, Elsevier Inc., 360 Park Avenue South, New York, New York 10010-1710. Tel. 212-633-3874, Fax: 212-633-3820, E-mail: reprints@elsevier.com.

The Surgical Clinics of North America is also published in Spanish by McGraw-Hill Interamericana Editores S.A., P.O. Box 5-237 06500 Mexico D.F. Mexico; and in Portuguese by Interlivros Edicoes Ltda., Rua Comandante Coelho 1085, CEP 21250, Rio de Janeiro, Brazil; and in Greek by Paschalidis Medical Publications, Athens Greece.

The Surgical Clinics of North America is covered in *MEDLINE/PubMed (Index Medicus), EMBASE/Excerpta Medica, Current Contents/Clinical Medicine, Current Contents/Life Sciences, Science Citation Index,* and *ISI/BIOMED.*

Contributors

CONSULTING EDITOR

RONALD F. MARTIN, MD, FACS
Colonel (ret.), United States Army Reserve, Department of Surgery, York Hospital, York, Maine

EDITOR

SUSHANTH REDDY, MD
Assistant Professor, Department of Surgery, School of Medicine, The University of Alabama at Birmingham, Birmingham, Alabama

AUTHORS

NITA AHUJA, MD, MBA
Department of Surgery, Yale University, School of Medicine, New Haven, Connecticut

CHANDRAKANTH ARE, MD, MBA
JL & CJ Varner Professor of Surgical Oncology and Global Health, Associate Dean of Graduate Medical Education (DIO), Vice Chair of Education, Department of Surgery, University of Nebraska Medical Center, Omaha, Nebraska

FEREDUN S. AZARI, MD
Department of Surgery, Hospital of the University of Pennsylvania, Philadelphia, Pennsylvania

RISHI BATRA, MD, MBA
General Surgery Resident, Department of Surgery, University of Nebraska Medical Center, Omaha, Nebraska

CARLO M. CONTRERAS, MD
Associate Professor, Department of Surgery, The University of Alabama at Birmingham, Birmingham, Alabama

MATTHEW R. EGYUD, MD
Department of Surgery, Boston University School of Medicine, Boston, Massachusetts

TONY E. GODFREY, PhD
Professor of Surgery and Computational Biomedicine, Department of Surgery, Boston University School of Medicine, Boston, Massachusetts

ALISON L. HALPERN, MD
General Surgery Residency, Department of Surgery, Division of Surgical Oncology, University of Colorado School of Medicine, Aurora, Colorado

RAJAT KUMAR, MD
Cardiothoracic Surgery Resident, Division of Cardiothoracic Surgery, Department of Surgery, The University of Alabama Birmingham Medical Center, Birmingham, Alabama

ANNE O. LIDOR, MD, MPH, FACS
Professor of Surgery, Chief, Division of Minimally Invasive and Bariatric Surgery, Department of Surgery, University of Wisconsin School of Medicine, Madison, Wisconsin

JAMES D. LUKETICH, MD
Henry T Bahnson Professor and Chairman, Department of Cardiothoracic Surgery, University of Pittsburgh Medical Center, University of Pittsburgh School of Medicine, University of Pittsburgh, Pittsburgh, Pennsylvania

GAUTAM K. MALHOTRA, MS, MD, PhD
General Surgery Resident, Department of Surgery, University of Nebraska Medical Center, Omaha, Nebraska

LAURA M. MAZER, MD, MS
Fellow, Division of Minimally Invasive Surgery, Cedars-Sinai Medical Center, Los Angeles, CA

IGOR WANKO MBOUMI, MD
Chief, Division of Minimally Invasive and Bariatric Surgery, Department of Surgery, University of Wisconsin School of Medicine, Madison, Wisconsin

MARTIN D. McCARTER, MD, FACS
Professor, Department of Surgery, Division of Surgical Oncology, University of Colorado School of Medicine, Aurora, Colorado

OMEED MOAVEN, MD
Instructor, Division of Surgical Oncology, Department of Surgery, Wake Forest University, Winston-Salem, North Carolina

NORMAN G. NICOLSON, MD
Department of Surgery, Yale University, School of Medicine, New Haven, Connecticut

ARJUN PENNATHUR, MD
Sampson Family Endowed Chair in Thoracic Surgical Oncology, Department of Cardiothoracic Surgery, University of Pittsburgh Medical Center, University of Pittsburgh School of Medicine, University of Pittsburgh, Pittsburgh, Pennsylvania

GEORGE A. POULTSIDES, MD, MS, FACS
Associate Professor, Section of Surgical Oncology, Stanford University School of Medicine, Stanford, California

SUSHANTH REDDY, MD
Assistant Professor, Department of Surgery, School of Medicine, The University of Alabama at Birmingham, Birmingham, Alabama

ROBERT E. ROSES, MD
Department of Surgery, Hospital of the University of Pennsylvania, Philadelphia, Pennsylvania

JILL C. RUBINSTEIN, MD, PhD
Department of Surgery, Yale University, School of Medicine, New Haven, Connecticut

SHAILENDER SINGH, MD
Associate Professor, Internal Medicine, Division of Gastroenterology-Hepatology, Omaha, Nebraska

KEI SUZUKI, MD
Department of Surgery, Boston University School of Medicine, Boston Medical Center, Boston, Massachusetts

LAUREN THEISS, MD
Department of Surgery, The University of Alabama at Birmingham, Birmingham, Alabama

JENNIFER F. TSENG, MD, MPH
Department of Surgery, Boston University School of Medicine, Boston Medical Center, Boston, Massachusetts

THOMAS N. WANG, MD, PhD
Professor, Department of Surgery, Division of Surgical Oncology, The University of Alabama at Birmingham, Birmingham, Alabama

BENJAMIN WEI, MD
Associate Professor, Division of Cardiothoracic Surgery, Department of Surgery, The University of Alabama Birmingham Medical Center, Birmingham, Alabama

Contents

Esophageal cancer and gastric cancer are leading causes of cancer-related mortality worldwide. In this article, the authors discuss the molecular biology of esophageal and gastric cancer with a focus on esophageal adenocarcinoma. They review data from The Cancer Genome Atlas project and advances in the molecular stratification and classification of esophageal carcinoma and gastric cancer. They also summarize advances in microRNA, molecular staging, gene expression profiling, tumor microenvironment, and detection of circulating tumor DNA. Finally, the authors summarize some of the implications of understanding the molecular basis of esophageal cancer and future directions in the management of esophageal cancer.

Multimodality therapy is the standard of care for locoregional esophageal cancers (greater than clinical T3 or Nb), including Siewert type 1 and 2 gastroesophageal junction tumors. Induction regimen, chemotherapy only or chemoradiation, is an area of controversy and often institution-specific, as neither has shown to be superior. Response to induction therapy is an important prognostic marker. For esophageal squamous cell carcinoma, it may be acceptable to observe clinical complete responders after chemoradiotherapy and perform salvage esophagectomy for recurrent disease. Clinical T2N0 esophageal cancer presents a unique challenge given its inaccuracy in clinical staging; management of this particular subset is controversial.

Esophageal and gastric carcinomas are prevalent malignancies worldwide. In contrast to the poor prognosis associated with advanced stages of disease, early stage disease has a favorable prognosis. Early stage gastric cancer (ESGC) is defined as cancer in which the depth of invasion is limited to the submucosal layer of the stomach on histologic examination, regardless of lymph node status. ESGC that meets standard or expanded criteria can be treated via endoscopic mucosal resection and endoscopic submucosal dissection. Similar indications for endoscopic interventions exist for gastroesophageal junction and esophageal malignancies.

Cancer of the gastroesophageal junction (GEJ) is increasing in incidence, likely as a result of rising obesity and gastroesophageal reflux disease rates. The tumors that arise here share features of esophageal and gastric cancer, and are classified based on their location in relationship to the GEJ. The definition of the GEJ itself, as well as optimal resection strategy, extent of lymph node dissection, resection margin length, and reconstruction methods are still very much a subject of debate. This article summarizes the available evidence on this topic, and highlights specific areas for further research.

A variety of esophageal diseases are treated with esophagectomy, from benign to esophageal cancer. Careful attention must be given to management of the difficult conduit, including patients who have had prior gastric surgery and other procedures, patients with conditions such as diabetic gastroparesis, which can affect the stomach as a future usable conduit, and patients who have an absent or unusable stomach. In these situations, consideration should be raised for the use of alternative conduits, including jejunal and colonic interposition conduits. The esophageal surgeon should also be adept at management of intraoperative difficulties with the conduit.

Human evolutionary genetic divergence and distinctive environmental exposures have contributed to the development of clinicopathologic variations of esophageal cancer in Eastern and Western countries. Different treatment strategies have derived from the disparate regional experiences. Treatment strategy is more standardized in the West. Trimodality treatment with neoadjuvant chemoradiation followed by surgery is widely accepted as the standard treatment of locally advanced esophageal adenocarcinoma and esophageal squamous cell carcinoma. Trimodality treatment has not been adopted in many Eastern countries, and standard treatment is neoadjuvant chemotherapy. Several randomized trials are ongoing that may alter the standard management of esophageal cancer worldwide.

Esophagectomy is the mainstay for treating esophageal cancers and other pathology. Even with refinements in surgical techniques and the introduction of minimally invasive approaches, the overall morbidity remains formidable. Complications, if not quickly recognized, can lead to significant long-term sequelae and even death. Vigilance with a high degree of suspicion remains the surgeon's greatest ally when caring for a patient who has recently undergone an esophagectomy. In this review, we highlight different

approaches in dealing with anastomotic leaks, chyle leaks, cardiopulmonary complications, and later functional issues after esophagectomy.

Jill C. Rubinstein, Norman G. Nicolson, and Nita Ahuja

Next-generation sequencing has enabled genome-wide molecular
profiling of gastric and esophageal malignancies at single-nucleotide resolution. The resultant genomic profiles provide information about the specific oncogenic pathways that are the likely driving forces behind
tumorigenesis and progression. The abundance of available genomic
data has immense potential to redefine management paradigms for these
difficult disease processes. The ability to capitalize on the information provided through high-throughput sequencing technologies will define cancer
care in the coming decades and could shift the paradigm from current
stage-based, organ-specific treatments toward tailored regimens that
target the specific culprit pathways driving individual tumors.

Rishi Batra, Gautam K. Malhotra, Shailender Singh, and Chandrakanth Are

This article reviews the pathophysiology, risk factors, clinical presentation/
diagnosis, and management of SCC.

Lauren Theiss and Carlo M. Contreras

Gastrointestinal stromal tumors (GISTs) arise anywhere along the gastrointestinal tract, most commonly as a result of c-kit or PDGFRA proto-
oncogene mutations. Surgical resection is an important component of
treatment. However, molecular profiling of GISTs has provided many in-
sights into adjuvant and neoadjuvant therapy options. Imatinib, the most
frequently studied medical therapy, has been shown in numerous studies
to provide benefit to patients in both the neoadjuvant and adjuvant setting.
Interval imaging is an important component of the treatment of GISTs and
national surveillance recommendations should be followed.

Alison L. Halpern and Martin D. McCarter

In patients with advanced esophageal or gastric cancer, it is highly likely that
palliation of symptoms will become a focus of treatment. Dysphagia and
obstruction are the most common complaints, and many of these patients
can be treated with endoscopic interventions to alleviate symptoms.
Bleeding, perforation, and nutritional issues are common problems. Attempts at palliation should be guided by thoughtful discussions regarding
patients' goals of care. Owing to the high morbidity and mortality in patients
with limited life expectancy, a strategy of working from the least invasive to
the most invasive interventions should be guided by the patient's goals.

SURGICAL CLINICS
OF NORTH AMERICA

SERIES OF RELATED INTEREST

Advances in Surgery
Available at: www.advancessurgery.com
Surgical Oncology Clinics
Available at: www.surgonc.theclinics.com
Thoracic Surgery Clinics
Available at: www.thoracic.theclinics.com

THE CLINICS ARE AVAILABLE ONLINE!
Access your subscription at:
www.theclinics.com

Foreword

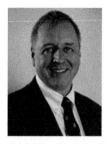

Ronald F. Martin, MD, FACS
Consulting Editor

For those of you who have followed this series for some time, you will most likely have noticed that much of the effort in our continued publishing at some level tries to address boundaries: frequently shifting boundaries. We try in our own way to consider the boundaries between general surgeons and specialty surgeons. We give pause to consider those efforts that can be delivered by few or must be delivered by many. We ponder the shifting roles of surgeons as leaders, collaborators, or even support players in multidisciplinary groups. Even within our domain as surgeons, we consider anatomic boundaries to our craft.

Some of the shifts in anatomic "domain" have lasted. Proctology has become colorectal surgery (and is unlikely to go back). Those surgeons who work on vessels have largely separated from those who work near vessels. One anatomic area has blurred substantially: the area of foregut surgery.

Foregut surgery means different things to different people. Some think bariatric/metabolic operations define foregut surgery. Others think antireflux and hiatal defect operations do, while others think resectional/reconstructive therapy for malignant disorders (or benign, I suppose) of the esophagus, stomach, duodenum, and pancreas defines the discipline. All of the people who hold the above opinions are right to some extent, and to some extent it doesn't really matter what we call it.

Most of us would acknowledge that the skill sets required to work in the peritoneal cavity, or the retroperitoneum, or the mediastinum, or either hemithorax are similar in some regards and dissimilar in others. When we add in the skill set layers to incorporate advanced technology as well as experience in recognizing normal and abnormal anatomy from multiple visual perspectives, we truly create a diverse set of tools that one has to master to do all of the foregut operations. Very few people actually do that.

This particular issue of the *Surgical Clinics of North America* was originally conceived to address a series of questions about these blurring of boundaries. In particular, how does our perspective and knowledge shape our thinking about malignancies that originate within a few centimeters of one another near the esophagogastric junction? At first, it would seem like a pretty mundane question, but after studying a bit, it gets pretty daunting.

Surg Clin N Am 99 (2019) xi–xii
https://doi.org/10.1016/j.suc.2019.03.002
0039-6109/19/© 2019 Published by Elsevier Inc.

For those who are truly nostalgic for the old days of Halstedian thought, perhaps we can just cut out everything in the area, hook up what is left, and hope it does not leak. For those who dream of a somewhat more utopian future, we will be able to obtain a few cells, and with precision medicine obliterate the problem or regress it to a nonmalignant state. For those us who must live in the present, the reality falls somewhere in between.

We do have better drugs. We do have better endoscopic options to resection. We do have operations that are better tailored to removing that which we must while preserving what we can. And, as with so many other diseases, we are better positioned to work with our colleagues who are not surgeons to help our patients pick and choose the best options. To do so, however, requires diligence and continued learning in a field that burgeons before us. To that end, we are deeply indebted to Dr Reddy and his colleagues for assembling this collection of articles to help our readership understand a very challenging and changing field.

I am reasonably confident that despite our years of discussing these topics through the *Surgical Clinics of North America*, we have raised more questions than we have provided answers for the boundary topics listed above. To be honest, that is what I had hoped for when I began doing this. Answers are great, and they have a certain value, no doubt. We all like to find them and are reassured when we have what we believe are answers. Our belief that we *know* something comforts us. Yet, most "definitive" answers eventually fail, but good questions always endure.

Most of us as surgeons have benefited from our predecessors having time or making time to ponder the big questions. Some of those questions took more than one career to work though. In today's environment, there aren't many relative value units associated with taking time for big picture thinking. We are very fortunate to have people left who can find time for inquiry and reflection. We are even more fortunate that so many of those people still share their ideas and knowledge with the rest of us.

Ronald F. Martin, MD, FACS
United States Army Reserve, retired
Department of Surgery
York Hospital
16 Hospital Drive, Suite A
York, ME 03909, USA

E-mail address:
rmartin@yorkhospital.com

Preface

Surgical Challenges of the Foregut

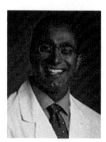

Sushanth Reddy, MD
Editor

As a student, I understood the gastrointestinal (GI) tract to be a single, long tubular structure with different names along the way. I thought, if any portion were to have pathology, that section could simply be removed, and the two ends brought back together to restore normal anatomy and function. My entire world was rocked to a core when I read about Cesar Roux and his attempt to prevent biliary reflux and marginal ulcers. Roux-en-Y reconstructions are now a mainstay of the gastric surgeon's toolbox.

Many of our surgical predecessors were wizards of gastric and esophageal surgery. With advances in antacid medications, the role of surgery in caring for benign ulcer diseases of the foregut has largely become footnotes in historical text. However, malignant diseases of the stomach and esophagus have become increasingly prevalent throughout the world. Surgical resection has consistently been the mainstay of esophageal, gastroesophageal (GE) junction, and gastric cancer therapy, and surgical management, from the workup to managing complications, should be in the armamentarium for the general surgeon. Modern technical consideration includes minimally invasive techniques, including laparoscopic and robotic removal of these tumors as well as complex endoscopic management. In addition, greater attention to patients' nutritional status has greatly reduced operative mortality and morbidity. Finally, surgical correction of GE reflux disease remains a common operation and can render management of these cancers far more complex.

Much of what we know about these cancers is derived from experiences from different parts of the world. Gastric adenocarcinoma is endemic in East Asia as is esophageal squamous cell carcinoma. However, esophageal and GE junction adenocarcinoma is seen primarily in Western populations. These basic findings introduce the genetic and epigenetic differences in these tumors' biology. Large prospective clinical trials for these cancers were conducted and published out of Europe; upfront systemic therapy is favored in Western populations, while surgery is the first-line therapy in Asia.

Surg Clin N Am 99 (2019) xiii–xiv
https://doi.org/10.1016/j.suc.2019.03.001
0039-6109/19/© 2019 Published by Elsevier Inc.

surgical.theclinics.com

Differences in epidemiology and tumor progression may account for different success rates of treatment approaches throughout the world. Gastrointestinal stromal tumors (GIST) were once thought to be rare, but they may be more common. In contrast to earlier tactics supporting an aggressive surgical approach, the development of biological therapy (including imatinib by surgeons) has shown us that not every GIST requires resection, and a multidisciplinary approach leads to better patient outcomes.

We discuss these topics in great detail in this issue of the *Surgical Clinics of North America*. I would like to personally thank each of the authors for contributing their effort toward this issue. The overall outcomes of these patients have greatly improved due to many of the advances discussed here; however, much remains to be discovered. None of the topics here comes to a complete conclusion, and I hope that readers become encouraged to explore the questions raised for future generations.

Sushanth Reddy, MD
Department of Surgery
School of Medicine
The University of Alabama at Birmingham
Birmingham, AL 35294, USA

E-mail address:
sreddy@uabmc.edu

The Molecular Biologic Basis of Esophageal and Gastric Cancers

Arjun Pennathur, MD[a],*, Tony E. Godfrey, PhD[b], James D. Luketich, MD[a]

KEYWORDS

- Esophageal cancer • Gastric cancer • Molecular biology • Gene expression
- Survival • MicroRNA • Tumor microenvironment • Molecular staging

KEY POINTS

- The Cancer Genome Atlas Project analysis proposed 4 molecular types of gastric cancer and 3 types of esophageal squamous cell carcinoma (ESCC). ESCC molecularly resembles other squamous cell cancers (lung and head and neck squamous cell cancer) more closely than it resembles esophageal adenocarcinoma (EAC).
- There are significant similarities between EAC and gastric adenocarcinoma with chromosomal instability (CIN), but EAC has more frequent hypermethylation than CIN gastric cancers.
- Gene expression profiles in EAC are significantly associated with patient outcomes.
- Investigation of the tumor microenvironment is an evolving area of research.
- The detection of circulating tumor DNA (ctDNA) is an active area of research, and ctDNA may play an important role in diagnosis, treatment monitoring, and management of esophageal cancer.

INTRODUCTION

Esophageal cancer and gastric cancer are leading causes of cancer-related mortality. The total annual incidence of esophageal and gastric cancer is more than 1.4 million worldwide, with more than 1.1 million deaths a year from these cancers.[1–3]

Disclosures: This work has been supported in part by NIH grants 5RO1 CA090665 09, R01CA208599, R01CA130853, R01CA130853 Supplement, 1R21CA172999, HHSN261201000058c, and P30CA047904. We would also like to acknowledge the support of a DeGregorio Family Foundation Research grant (TEG) and a University of Pittsburgh Physicians (UPP) Foundation grant, the University of Pittsburgh Sampson Family Endowed Chair, and the Jane France and Chris Allison philanthropic grant support.

[a] Department of Cardiothoracic Surgery, University of Pittsburgh Medical Center, The University of Pittsburgh School of Medicine, University of Pittsburgh, 200 Lothrop St. Suite C-800, Pittsburgh, PA 15213, USA; [b] Department of Surgery, Boston University School of Medicine, 700 Albany St, Boston, MA 02118, USA
* Corresponding author.
E-mail address: pennathura@upmc.edu

Surg Clin N Am 99 (2019) 403–418
https://doi.org/10.1016/j.suc.2019.02.010
0039-6109/19/© 2019 Elsevier Inc. All rights reserved.
surgical.theclinics.com

Esophageal cancer affects more than 450,000 people worldwide, and the incidence of esophageal cancer is rapidly increasing.[4,5] The incidence of each type of esophageal and gastric cancer varies geographically. In this article, the authors review the epidemiology, risk factors, and molecular biology of esophageal and gastric tumors with a focus on esophageal adenocarcinoma (EAC).

An accumulation of molecular alterations in the genome of the somatic cell is the molecular basis of cancer.[6] The rapid advances in DNA sequencing technology have significantly improved the understanding of cancer molecular biology and will continue to have an impact in the future. The potential effects of advances in molecular technology include redesigning tumor taxonomy from a histology- or anatomy-based classification to a molecular-based classification, personalized treatment based on specific therapies that target the molecular changes driving tumorigenesis, gene profiling to assist with individualized treatment and identification of tumor-specific mutations, and "liquid biopsies" of blood samples for detection of cancer and monitoring of therapy.[6]

In this review, the authors discuss the findings of The Cancer Genome Atlas (TCGA) research group and others describing molecular changes in esophageal and gastric cancer.[7–10] They summarize recent advances in the molecular classification of esophageal carcinoma, molecular similarities and differences between EAC and gastric cancer, molecular stratification of esophageal squamous cell carcinoma (ESCC), and similarities with other squamous cell carcinomas. In addition, the authors summarize some recent work on microRNA (miRNA) in the differentiation of Barrett esophagus (BE) and esophageal carcinoma, the prognostic value of miRNA and gene expression profiles in EAC, tumor microenvironment, and recent advances in circulating tumor DNA (ctDNA) in the diagnosis and management of esophageal cancer.[11–22] Finally, the authors summarize some of the implications of understanding the molecular basis of esophageal cancer, and future directions in the management of esophageal cancer.

ESOPHAGEAL CARCINOMA: EPIDEMIOLOGY AND RISK FACTORS

ESCC is the most common type of esophageal cancer worldwide; however, there has been a striking shift in the epidemiology of esophageal cancer in western countries, with the incidence of EAC now exceeding that of ESCC.[23–25] The rate of this increase in the incidence of EAC has been quite dramatic, particularly in Caucasians. The cause of this increase is not clear; however, as described in later discussion, it is associated with gastroesophageal reflux disease (GERD), obesity, and BE.[1] The rising incidence in the United States is not due to either overdiagnosis or reclassification of esophageal carcinoma based on histology or location.[25] Other less-common types of esophageal cancer include melanoma, leiomyosarcoma, and small cell carcinoma.[23]

Tobacco use has been associated with both ESCC and EAC and is thought to be related to exposure to nitrosamines.[26] Alcohol consumption is risk factor for ESCC but does not appear to be a risk factor for EAC.[27,28] The pathophysiology appears to involve a metabolite of alcohol, aldehyde, which is a carcinogen. Mutations affecting enzymes that metabolize alcohol increase the risk of ESCC.[29] Achalasia and caustic injury are additional risk factors for ESCC, and a history of thoracic radiation is a risk factor for both ESCC and EAC.[23,30] ESCC is also associated with a lower socioeconomic status and nutritional deficiencies, such as Plummer-Vinson syndrome.[23,31]

In the United States, ESCC is predominantly associated with smoking and alcohol consumption, whereas in developing countries, other factors, such as nutritional deficiencies (vitamin E, selenium, zinc), and oral hygiene are associated with ESCC.[32–34] Nonepidermolytic palmoplantar keratoderma (tylosis), an autosomal dominant disorder, with mutation of the gene RHBDF2, is associated with a high risk for ESCC, and genetic polymorphisms that are associated with ESCC have also been described, including TP53 mutation.[35,36]

The major risk factors for EAC include symptomatic GERD, obesity, BE, cigarette smoking, and a diet that is low in vegetables and fruits.[37,38] BE is a condition that is strongly associated with EAC, wherein the esophageal squamous mucosa is replaced by specialized columnar epithelium. The risk of a patient with BE developing EAC is estimated to be 0.5% per year, with the highest risk in patients with high-grade dysplasia (HGD) of the esophagus.[1,39]

GASTRIC CANCER: EPIDEMIOLOGY AND RISK FACTORS

As seen for esophageal cancer, there are geographic variations in the incidence of gastric cancer, with an increasing incidence of adenocarcinoma of the gastric cardia and gastroesophageal junction in Western countries. In contrast, noncardia gastric adenocarcinoma is more prevalent in Asia, Africa, Eastern Europe, and South America.[2,3] Most gastric cancers are of adenocarcinoma histology; however, gastric adenocarcinoma is very heterogeneous.[2] As per the Lauren classification scheme, gastric cancers can be separated into 2 main types: intestinal types, which are primarily moderately differentiated, and diffuse types, which are predominantly poorly differentiated; other types include mixed and indeterminate types. Another classification used by the World Health Organization (WHO) includes 5 main categories based on histologic patterns. WHO categories of tubular and papillary correlate with the Lauren intestinal type, and the poorly cohesive WHO type corresponds to the diffuse Lauren type.[2]

Helicobacter pylori bacterial infection is the most commonly associated risk factor with sporadic gastric cancer.[40] Epstein-Barr virus (EBV) is also associated with gastric cancer.[41,42] Hereditary gastric cancer accounts for ~1% to 3% of all gastric cancers, and mutations in CDH1 and CTNNA1 have been identified in hereditary diffuse cancers.[43] Gastric cancers have also been found in hereditary cancer syndromes, such as Li-Fraumeni syndrome, which is characterized by mutations in TP53.[2,43] Similar to esophageal cancer, risk factors for gastric cancer include a diet low in fruits and vegetables, smoking, and obesity.[2,44–46] GERD and obesity are associated with an increasing incidence of gastroesophageal junction adenocarcinoma.[25]

MOLECULAR CHARACTERIZATION OF ESOPHAGEAL CARCINOMA

Because of the striking epidemiologic differences between ESCC and EAC, the authors and their collaborators investigated genomic differences between these 2 histologic subtypes, which could be important for developing new therapeutic strategies for esophageal cancer.[13] The authors explored DNA copy number abnormalities using single nucleotide polymorphism arrays in 259 esophageal tumors (70 ESCC and 189 EAC). In this analysis, the authors found that ESCC and EAC showed some copy number abnormalities with similar frequencies (eg, CDKN2A, EGFR, KRAS, MYC, CDK6, MET, MCL1, SMURF1, ERBB2, CCNE1, VEGFA, and IGF1R.) Of these, EGFR, ERBB2, VEGFA, and MET are targets of currently available therapeutic agents. There were also many copy number abnormalities with different frequencies between the 2 histologic types. Genes with different amplification frequencies between ESCC and EAC included SOX2, PIK3CA, MYC, CCND1, FGFR1, GATA4, and GATA6. One of the most striking differences observed was amplification of 3q (60% of ESCC vs

15% of EAC), which contains both SOX2 and PIK3CA. SOX2 has been implicated as a lineage-specific oncogene for squamous cell tumors.[47] Most of these differences were amplification events. Some of these regions harbor genes that are possible targets for therapy, including PIK3CA and FGFR1. The authors concluded from this study using single nucleotide polymorphism arrays that there were both similar and different copy number abnormalities in ESCC and EAC, which may allow for development of histology-specific targeted therapies in esophageal cancer.

The authors participated in another multi-institutional study of whole-exome sequencing in 149 patients with EAC; 15 patients also had whole-genome sequencing analysis.[8] The mutational signature had high A > C transitions at AA dinucleotides. The authors found 26 significantly mutated genes in EAC (false discovery rate q <0.1), with TP53 and CDKN2A being most significant. Other known mutations included SMAD4, ARID1A, and PIK3CA. In addition, new significant mutations found included SPG20, TLR4, ELMO1, and DOCK2. In this analysis, there was high mutation frequency in EAC with a median mutation rate of 9.9 mutations/megabase (which is higher than colorectal cancer, where the median mutation frequency was 5.6 mutations/megabase). In addition, mutations in chromosomal remodeling enzymes were found. Lawrence and colleagues[48] analyzed multiple cancers and found that the mutational load in esophageal and gastric tumors was high (**Fig. 1**). This high mutational load may indicate that these tumors might be responsive to immunotherapy.[3,49]

THE CANCER GENOME ATLAS MOLECULAR CHARACTERIZATION OF ESOPHAGEAL CARCINOMA AND COMPARISON WITH GASTRIC CARCINOMA

In one of the largest and most comprehensive analyses of esophageal cancer, the authors participated in a multicenter collaborative research effort: TCGA, a landmark cancer genomics program coordinated by the National Institutes of Health (NIH).[10] In this study, TCGA investigators published the integrated genomic characterization of esophageal cancer with a comprehensive molecular analysis of 164 esophageal tumors (ESSC, n = 90; EAC, n = 72; undifferentiated, n = 2), 359 gastric tumors, and 36 adenocarcinomas of the gastroesophageal junction. This comprehensive analysis

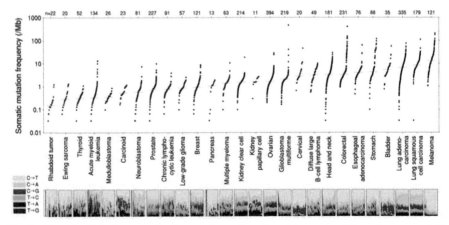

Fig. 1. Mutational heterogeneity in esophageal and gastric cancer. (*From* Lawrence MS, Stojanov P, Polak P, et al. Mutational heterogeneity in cancer and the search for new cancer-associated genes. Nature 2013;499(7457):214–218; with permission from Springer Nature.)

included whole-exome sequencing, single nucleotide polymorphism profiling to detect somatic copy number alternations (SCNA), DNA methylation, messenger RNA (mRNA), and miRNA sequencing.

Gene Expression Analysis

In TCGA project investigations, gene expression analysis showed that EACs have increased in E-cadherin expression and upregulation of pathways that regulate E-cadherin. ESCCs showed upregulation of Wnt, syndecan, and p63 pathways. This differential expression suggests that different alterations may drive the progression of ESCC and EAC.

Somatic Genomic Alterations

Somatic alterations were evaluated to search for genes with recurring mutations. In EAC, there were significant mutations noted in TP53, CDKN2A, ARID1A, SMAD4, and ERBB2. Notably, TP53 and CDKN2A were shown in previous studies to harbor mutations in BE as well.[8] Furthermore, as described in later discussion, the authors have also found that CDKN2A gene expression is part of a gene expression signature predictive of survival in EAC.[11] In ESCC, mutations of TP53, NFE2L2, MLL2, ZNF750, NOTCH1, and TGFBR2 were found.

Combined Mutation and Somatic Copy Number Alternations Data

Frequent alterations were noted in cell-cycle regulators in TCGA project analyses, and the patterns of alteration of SCNAs differed between ESSC and EAC. In ESCC, inactivation of CDKN2A was noted in 76% and amplification of CCND1 was noted in 57%. In EAC, CDKN2A was inactivated in 76%, similar to ESCC, but CCND1 was amplified less frequently (15% for EAC vs 57% for ESCC). These data suggest a potential role for targeting cell-cycle kinases in the treatment of esophageal cancer.

Molecular Subtypes of Esophageal Squamous Cell Cancer

In an interesting integrative clustering analysis of the ESCC data, was classified into 3 molecular subtypes in TCGA project analyses. ESCC cluster 1 (n = 50) had alterations in the NRF2 pathway, which have been associated with resistance to chemoradiation and worse prognosis.[10,40] They also had a higher frequency of SOX2 and TP63 amplification. The gene expression of ESCC cluster 1 resembled the classical subtype described in TCGA lung squamous cell cancer and head and neck squamous cell cancer. ESCC cluster 2 (n = 36) showed mutations in NOTCH 1 and ZNF750 mutations. ESCC cluster 3 (n = 4) had PI3K gene alternations predicted to activate the PI3K pathway and did not resemble head and neck SCC, suggesting that this type may be limited to ESCC. TP53 mutations were present in only one sample in ESCC cluster 3. Geographic variations in the incidence of these subtypes were noted. ESCC from Asia tended to be ESCC subtype 1 (27/41%; 66%), and all 4 samples with ESCC subtype 3 were from the United States and Canada. Eastern European and South American samples tended to be of the ESSC subtype 2. Combined analysis of mRNA, DNA methylation, and SCNA from ESCC revealed that ESCC had a stronger resemblance to head and neck squamous cell cancer than to EAC.

GASTRIC CARCINOMA: THE CANCER GENOME ATLAS ANALYSIS

The authors participated in a multicenter collaborative TCGA research effort to comprehensively characterize the molecular alterations in gastric adenocarcinoma.[9] A total of 295 patient samples, collected from centers worldwide, were analyzed in this comprehensive analysis. Six platforms were used for molecular characterization, including SCNA, whole-exome sequencing, DNA methylation profiling, mRNA, and miRNA sequencing, and reverse phase protein arrays. From this comprehensive analysis, 4 major genomic subtypes of gastric cancer were described (**Fig. 2**): (1) EBV-infected tumors, (2) Tumors with microsatellite instability (MSI), (3) Genomically stable (GS) tumors, and (4) Tumors with chromosomally instability (CIN). The EBV-positive tumors (9%) had recurring mutations of PIK3CA, extreme hypermethylation, and amplification of JAK2, PD-L1, and PD-L2. The tumors with MSI (22%) showed increased mutation rates particularly in the genes for oncogenic signaling proteins. The GS tumors (20%) were enriched for the diffuse histology subtype and had mutations in the Rho family, and tumors with CIN (50%) showed marked aneuploidy and focal amplification of tyrosine kinases. Notably, the CIN tumors were predominant (65%) in the gastroesophageal junction and the gastric cardia, whereas the EBV-positive tumors (62%) were primarily noted in the fundus and body of the stomach.

Comparison of the Molecular Characteristics of Esophageal Adenocarcinoma and Gastric Adenocarcinoma

The molecular characteristics of EAC have been compared with the molecular characteristics of gastric carcinoma. As described above, TCGA analysis supported 4 subtypes of gastric carcinoma: EBV-infection, MSI, CIN, and GS, which was predominantly present in the diffuse histology subtype of gastric carcinoma. Interestingly, EAC resembled CIN gastric tumors, distinct from other subtypes. Notably, no EACs resembled the MSI or EBV gastric tumor subtypes, and 71 out of 72 gastroesophageal tumors were classified as CIN. Although there was a strong similarity in the

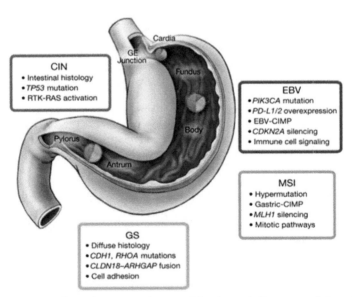

Fig. 2. Key features of gastric cancer subtypes. This schematic lists some of the salient features associated with each of the 4 molecular subtypes of gastric cancer. Distribution of molecular subtypes in tumors obtained from distinct regions of the stomach is represented by inset charts. CIMP, CpG island methylator phenotype; GE, gastroesophageal. (*From* Cancer Genome Atlas Research N. Comprehensive molecular characterization of gastric adenocarcinoma. Nature 2014;513(7517):202–209; with permission from Springer Nature.)

chromosomal aberrations between gastric CIN and EAC, there were also important differences in the DNA methylation. The proportion of cancers showing more frequent hypermethylation was significantly higher in EACs than in gastric cancers with CIN (70% vs 30%; $P = 1 \times 10^{-8}$).

In summary, TCGA analysis of ESCC, EAC, and gastric cancers showed distinct molecular characteristics similar to prior studies. ESCC resembles more closely squamous cell carcinoma from other sites (eg, head and neck cancer and lung squamous cell carcinoma). There were also striking similarities between EAC and CIN-type gastric cancer; however, there were also important differences in methylation between EAC and gastric adenocarcinoma. This comprehensive analysis may provide the framework for further molecular characterization of esophageal and gastric tumors and the development of more personalized targeted therapies that can be used in a neoadjuvant or adjuvant setting for the treatment of esophageal and gastric cancer.

MicroRNA, BARRETT ESOPHAGUS, AND ESOPHAGEAL CANCER

miRNAs are small noncoding RNA molecules and are posttranscriptional regulators of gene expression.[15,50] They regulate various cellular functions, including cell differentiation, proliferation, and apoptosis, and may function as either oncogenes or tumor suppressor genes. These miRNAs that are associated with cancer are collectively called oncomiRs.[15,51] The authors have previously reported the results of their collaborative study evaluating the miRNA expression in BE and esophageal cancer to identify potential markers for disease progression.[15] MiRNA expression patterns distinguish EAC, ESCC, normal squamous epithelium, BE, and HGD (**Fig. 3**). They found that miRNA expression may prove useful for identifying patients with BE at high risk for progression to EAC. Abnormalities in the mucosa in patients with BE, including chromosomal instability, the presence of aneuploidy/tetraploidy, and cell-cycle abnormalities, and p53 and Ki67 staining, are potential biomarkers for progression.[52,53] In a subsequent study, the authors evaluated the association of miRNA with

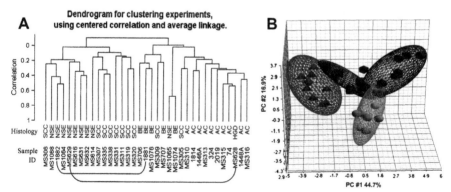

Fig. 3. MiRNA expression patterns distinguish esophageal adenocarcinoma (AC), squamous cell carcinoma (SCC), normal squamous epithelium (NSE), BE, and HGD. (*A*) Unsupervised hierarchical clustering of esophageal specimens with all expressed miRNAs. Linked samples (1882/1881 and MS629/MS628) were obtained from the same patient. (*B*) Principal component (PC) analysis mapping based on 14 miRNAs that exhibit differential expression between adenocarcinoma (*red triangle*), squamous cell carcinoma (*yellow circle*), normal squamous epithelium (*purple hexagon*), BE (*blue square*), and HGD (*green diamond*). (*From* Feber A, Xi L, Luketich JD, et al. MicroRNA expression profiles of esophageal cancer. J Thorac Cardiovasc Surg 2008;135(2):255–260; [discussion: 260]; with permission.)

lymph node metastases and survival in 45 patients with EAC.[54] They were able to identify a combined miRNA expression signature that was associated with patient survival ($P = .005$; hazard ratio 3.6) independent of node involvement and overall stage. They also found that the expression of 3 miRNAs was associated with the presence of lymph node metastasis.

This study suggests that miRNA expression profiling may provide additional value in staging EAC and predicting patient prognosis. Larger studies are required to fully evaluate the value of miRNA in esophageal cancer.

GENE EXPRESSION PROFILES PREDICT SURVIVAL IN PATIENTS WITH ESOPHAGEAL ADENOCARCINOMA

Gene expression profiling is a powerful and promising modality for evaluating the expression of a large number of genes and changes in their expression genome wide.[11,55,56] As described above, there are differences in the molecular makeup of esophageal tumors as well as similarities between esophageal tumors and a certain subtype of gastric cancer. The authors investigated the prognostic significance of gene expression profiling in 64 patients with EAC who underwent esophagectomy.[11] They applied unsupervised hierarchical clustering with 59 genes to construct a risk classifier and initially divided the 64-patient cohort into 2 clusters. This grouping successfully stratified patients by survival into low-risk (group A) and high-risk (group B) groups based on gene expression signature. High-risk patients had a predicted median survival of 19 months, whereas the median was not reached for the low-risk group ($P<.05$) (**Fig. 4**).

A risk score was calculated for each patient using 3 principal components for the 59 genes and was then divided into two risk groups to classify the patients. Analysis with Kaplan-Meier plots of these two groups (**Fig. 5**A) also demonstrated successful classification ($P = 7 \times 10^{-8}$). Notably, among the 32 patients identified as "low risk," only 7 deaths were observed as compared with 27 deaths of the 32 patients in the high-risk group. To assess the level of optimism in this estimate, the authors conducted repeated 10-fold cross-validation, 100 times. **Fig. 5**B shows that the cross-validated, high-risk group by gene expression signature had a significantly different

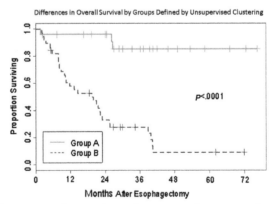

Differences in Overall Survival by Groups Defined by Unsupervised Clustering

$p<.0001$

Group A
Group B

Months After Esophagectomy

Fig. 4. Survival of patients with EAC who underwent esophagectomy classified into low-risk (group A) and high-risk (group B) groups by gene expression profiling. (*From* Pennathur A, Xi L, Litle VR, et al. Gene expression profiles in esophageal adenocarcinoma predict survival after resection. J Thorac Cardiovasc Surg 2013;145(2):505–512; [discussion: 512–513]; with permission.)

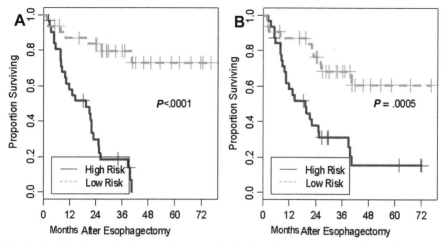

Fig. 5. Classification of patients with supervised principal components analysis. Three principal components were used to estimate a risk score for each patient according to their expression of the 59 genes. The risk score was divided into 2 groups at the median. (*A*) Comparison of low- and high-risk patient cohorts (*P*<.0001). (*B*) Same classification, using average of 100, 10-fold cross-validations to derive the risk score (*P* = .0005). (*From* Pennathur A, Xi L, Litle VR, et al. Gene expression profiles in esophageal adenocarcinoma predict survival after resection. J Thorac Cardiovasc Surg 2013;145(2):505–512; [discussion: 512–513]; with permission.)

overall survival than the group with the low-risk signature (*P* = .0005). Notably, 32% (8/ 25) of the T1 tumors studied had the high-risk gene expression signature associated with a worse prognosis.

This gene signature for risk classification was tested for significant association in a multivariate proportional hazards model that included pathologic T stage and N stage. A multivariate model of risk, after adjusting for both T and N stage, showed that the gene expression signature was independently associated with survival. The adjusted hazard ratio for the high-risk gene signature group was significant with a hazard ratio of 2.22 (95% confidence interval 1.02–4.03, *P* = .04) (**Fig. 6**).

An analysis of the pathways that are associated with this gene signature showed that the networks involved included those responsible for cellular assembly and reorganization, cell differentiation, cell proliferation, cell death, and inflammatory responses. One of the significantly associated cell-cycle genes was CDKN2A (cyclin-dependent kinase inhibitor 2A), which encodes p16 and acts through interaction with cyclin-dependent kinase-4.[11,57,58]

In summary, in this prospective study of patients with EAC treated with esophagectomy, the authors identified a preliminary, internally cross-validated 59-gene prognostic signature that was predictive of outcome in patients undergoing resection for EAC. If further validated, these results may help direct further clinical trials of neoadjuvant and adjuvant therapies for EAC.

TUMOR MICROENVIRONMENT AND STROMAL CONTRIBUTION

In addition to the tumor cells, the tumor microenvironment is also important in progression of cancer.[19,20,22] The tumor microenvironment comprises not only the cancer cells but also the extracellular matrix and other cells, including inflammatory cells,

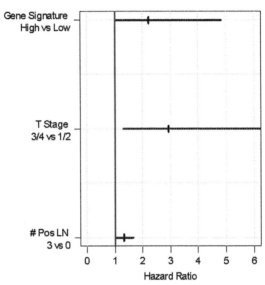

Fig. 6. Multivariate analysis. Red vertical line depicts hazard ratio of 1, indicating no effect. All factors remained significant at *P*<.05. Hazard ratio for gene signature, adjusting for T stage and N stage, was 2.2. (*From* Pennathur A, Xi L, Litle VR, et al. Gene expression profiles in esophageal adenocarcinoma predict survival after resection. J Thorac Cardiovasc Surg 2013;145(2):505–512; [discussion: 512–513]; with permission.)

immune cells, and fibroblasts.[20,21] The tumor microenvironment also has important implications in the immunology of cancer.[19] Cancer-related fibroblasts (CAFs) are an important component of tumor microenvironment, contribute to the mechanical properties of the stroma, and impact the secretion of cytokines.[21,22] Recently, Ebbing and colleagues[22] investigated the impact of stromal CAFs in EAC using patient-derived CAFs. They reported that interleukin-6 (IL-6) secreted by CAFs, activated an epithelial-to-mesenchymal transition in cancer cells and was identified as the stromal driver of therapy resistance in EAC. Interestingly, analysis of patient gene expression profiles identified ADAM12 as a serum biomarker for IL-6 secreting CAFs and was associated with decreased response to chemoradiation. This study demonstrates the importance of the stromal contribution to therapy resistance in EAC.

MOLECULAR STAGING OF LYMPH NODE METASTASES IN ESOPHAGEAL CANCER

The presence or absence of nodal metastases is one of the most important prognostic factors for survival in patients with esophageal cancer.[59] However, despite improvements in the clinical staging modalities, clinical nodal staging can still be inaccurate.[60–62] The staging of lymph nodes by molecular detection of markers with quantitative reverse-transcription polymerase chain reaction (qRT-PCR) may increase sensitivity in detecting lymph nodes positive for micrometastasis. Several studies have explored the prognostic significance of micrometastatic disease in ESCC; however, there are limited prospective studies evaluating the prognostic implications of micrometastasis in EAC.[63,64] The authors have previously evaluated molecular markers of micrometastasis in lymph nodes in EAC and found a panel of markers of potential prognostic significance.[63] They evaluated 39 markers initially; 6 underwent further analysis, and 5 were selected for an external validation study: CEA, CK7, TACSTD1,

CK19, and Villin 1. Two markers, TACSTD1 and CK19, provided excellent classification. The authors analyzed 34 patients with EAC and found that the disease-free survival was significantly worse in patients with positive nodes by molecular staging with multimarker qRT-PCR analysis (P = .0023). The detection of occult lymph node metastases appears to be more sensitive with qRT-PCR of selected markers than with standard detection methods, and larger prospective studies are needed to fully evaluate its value and prognostic significance.

CIRCULATING TUMOR DNA

An emerging area of interest in tumor molecular biology is the noninvasive detection of specific mutations with "liquid biopsy" of the serum or plasma via detection of ctDNA. The amount of cell-free DNA in the circulation is low (typically <20 ng/mL), and the fraction of ctDNA, particularly from an early-stage tumor, can be very low (<0.1%).[16,17] The detection of these tumor-specific mutations, therefore, can be challenging, because mutant allele fractions are low and represent only a small fraction of circulating, cell-free DNA. Jackson and colleagues[16] reported a multiplexed, preamplification step using a high-fidelity polymerase before digital PCR was developed to increase total DNA and used this method to detect multiple cancer-relevant mutations within tumor-derived samples down to 0.01%. More recently, barcoding of DNA template molecules early in next-generation sequencing (NGS) library construction has been described to identify and remove polymerase errors using bioinformatics. Stahlberg and colleagues[17] reported simple, multiplexed, PCR-based barcoding of DNA for sensitive mutation detection using sequencing to generate targeted barcoded libraries with minimal DNA input, flexible target selection, and a short library construction protocol. In an ongoing study, the authors are using this approach to evaluate ctDNA as a biomarker for diagnosis and monitoring of treatment for EAC. Recent preliminary investigations suggest that ctDNA levels in EAC patients correlate with response to therapy and that ctDNA can be detected in patients prior to clinical or radiographic evidence of recurrence.[65] Kato and colleagues[18] evaluated ctDNA from the plasma of 55 patients with gastroesophageal adenocarcinoma (mostly advanced stage) using NGS with a 54 to 73 gene panel. They found that 76% of patients (42/55) had ≥1 genomic alterations. The median number of alterations per patient was 2 (range, 0–15). The genes most frequently affected by the characterized alterations were TP53 (50.9%, 28/55), PIK3CA (16.4%, 9/55), ERBB2 (14.5%, 8/55), and KRAS (14.5%, 8/55) genes. The investigators also reported that ERBB2 alterations were significantly associated with poor overall survival. This study demonstrates that evaluation of ctDNA by NGS in patients with gastroesophageal adenocarcinoma is feasible.

IMPLICATIONS AND FUTURE DIRECTIONS

Molecular characterization of tumors, including gene expression profiling of the primary tumor, can provide useful information toward the understanding of the biological behavior of the tumor and personalized selection and tailoring of therapy. Gene expression signatures have the potential to significantly add to traditional clinical risk factors in the prediction of patient outcomes.[11] These findings, if validated, could lead to clinical trials based on the molecular characteristics of the primary tumor. Molecular staging in esophageal cancer has the potential to change treatment paradigms. Furthermore, the molecular characterization of primary esophageal and gastric tumors will allow us to develop personalized treatments that are specific and targeted based on the molecular makeup of a patient's tumor. The implications of

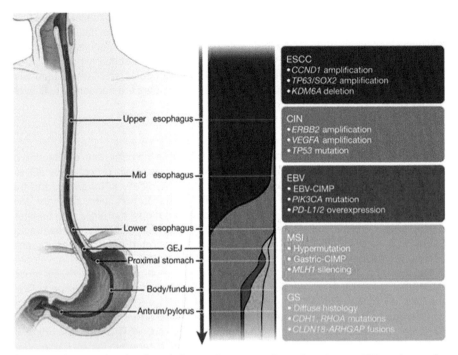

Fig. 7. Gradations of molecular subclasses of gastroesophageal carcinoma. GEJ, gastroesophageal junction. (*From* Cancer Genome Atlas Research N, Analysis Working Group: Asan U, Agency BCC, et al. Integrated genomic characterization of oesophageal carcinoma. Nature 2017;541(7636):169–175; used under the terms of the Creative Commons Attribution License [CC BY].)

NGS are described in more detail in Jill C. Rubinstein and colleagues' article, "Next Generation Sequencing in the Management of Gastric and Esophageal Cancers," in this issue. In addition, newer noninvasive modalities, such as "liquid biopsy" that evaluates ctDNA, may allow early detection of esophageal and gastric cancers, better monitoring of response to treatment, early detection of recurrent disease, and personalized treatment based on specific mutations noted in the tumor.

SUMMARY

Rapid advances in molecular biology technologies have significantly improved the understanding of esophageal and gastric cancer, including the ability to improve tumor taxonomy from a histology- or anatomy-based diagnosis to a molecular classification. It will also allow personalized treatment with specific therapies targeting the molecular changes driving tumorigenesis and gene profiling to assist with individualizing treatment. Molecular profiling of ESCC, EAC, and gastric cancers has revealed similarities and differences important to understanding the biology of these tumors (**Fig. 7**). ESCC molecularly resembles other squamous cell cancers more than it resembles EAC. There are significant similarities between EAC and the CIN type of gastric cancer. However, there are also significant differences between the two, with EAC being more frequently hypermethylated than CIN gastric cancers. The gene expression profiles of EAC are significantly associated with survival outcomes. The role of the tumor microenvironment is an evolving area of research. Furthermore, the detection of ctDNA is an active area of research with recent advances and may play an important role in the management of esophageal cancer.

ACKNOWLEDGMENTS

The authors acknowledge all our collaborators who contributed to this work, including collaborators in the NIH-sponsored TCGA network. We acknowledge the work of numerous investigators on esophageal and gastric cancer, who we were not able to cite due to limitations in size of the manuscript. The authors wish to thank and acknowledge the sincere efforts of our entire research team.

REFERENCES

1. Pennathur A, Gibson MK, Jobe BA, et al. Oesophageal carcinoma. Lancet 2013; 381(9864):400–12.
2. Van Cutsem E, Sagaert X, Topal B, et al. Gastric cancer. Lancet 2016;388(10060): 2654–64.
3. Lordick F, Janjigian YY. Clinical impact of tumour biology in the management of gastroesophageal cancer. Nat Rev Clin Oncol 2016;13(6):348–60.
4. Ferlay J, Shin HR, Bray F, et al. Estimates of worldwide burden of cancer in 2008: GLOBOCAN 2008. Int J Cancer 2010;127(12):2893–917.
5. Jemal A, Siegel R, Ward E, et al. Cancer statistics, 2009. CA Cancer J Clin 2009; 59(4):225–49.
6. DeVita VT, Lawrence TS, Rosenberg SA. Devita, Hellman, and Rosenberg's cancer: principles & practice of oncology. 11th edition. Philadelphia: Wolters Kluwer; 2018.
7. Dulak AM, Schumacher SE, van Lieshout J, et al. Gastrointestinal adenocarcinomas of the esophagus, stomach, and colon exhibit distinct patterns of genome instability and oncogenesis. Cancer Res 2012;72(17):4383–93.
8. Dulak AM, Stojanov P, Peng S, et al. Exome and whole-genome sequencing of esophageal adenocarcinoma identifies recurrent driver events and mutational complexity. Nat Genet 2013;45(5):478–86.
9. Cancer Genome Atlas Research Network. Comprehensive molecular characterization of gastric adenocarcinoma. Nature 2014;513(7517):202–9.
10. Cancer Genome Atlas Research Network, Analysis Working Group: Asan University, BC Cancer Agency, et al. Integrated genomic characterization of oesophageal carcinoma. Nature 2017;541(7636):169–75.
11. Pennathur A, Xi L, Litle VR, et al. Gene expression profiles in esophageal adenocarcinoma predict survival after resection. J Thorac Cardiovasc Surg 2013; 145(2):505–12 [discussion: 512–3].
12. Dong S, Zhao J, Wei J, et al. F-box protein complex FBXL19 regulates TGFbeta1-induced E-cadherin down-regulation by mediating Rac3 ubiquitination and degradation. Mol Cancer 2014;13:76.
13. Bandla S, Pennathur A, Luketich JD, et al. Comparative genomics of esophageal adenocarcinoma and squamous cell carcinoma. Ann Thorac Surg 2012;93(4): 1101–6.
14. Korkut A, Zaidi S, Kanchi RS, et al. A pan-cancer analysis reveals high-frequency genetic alterations in mediators of signaling by the TGF-beta superfamily. Cell Syst 2018;7(4):422–37.e7.
15. Feber A, Xi L, Luketich JD, et al. MicroRNA expression profiles of esophageal cancer. J Thorac Cardiovasc Surg 2008;135(2):255–60 [discussion: 260].

16. Jackson JB, Choi DS, Luketich JD, et al. Multiplex preamplification of serum DNA to facilitate reliable detection of extremely rare cancer mutations in circulating DNA by digital PCR. J Mol Diagn 2016;18(2):235–43.

17. Stahlberg A, Krzyzanowski PM, Egyud M, et al. Simple multiplexed PCR-based barcoding of DNA for ultrasensitive mutation detection by next-generation sequencing. Nat Protoc 2017;12(4):664–82.

18. Kato S, Okamura R, Baumgartner JM, et al. Analysis of circulating tumor DNA and clinical correlates in patients with esophageal, gastroesophageal junction, and gastric adenocarcinoma. Clin Cancer Res 2018;24(24):6248–56.

19. Joyce JA, Fearon DT. T cell exclusion, immune privilege, and the tumor microenvironment. Science 2015;348(6230):74–80.

20. Sun Y. Translational horizons in the tumor microenvironment: harnessing breakthroughs and targeting cures. Med Res Rev 2015;35(2):408–36.

21. Kalluri R, Zeisberg M. Fibroblasts in cancer. Nat Rev Cancer 2006;6(5):392–401.

22. Ebbing EA, van der Zalm AP, Steins A, et al. Stromal-derived interleukin 6 drives epithelial-to-mesenchymal transition and therapy resistance in esophageal adenocarcinoma. Proc Natl Acad Sci U S A 2019;116(6):2237–42.

23. Enzinger PC, Mayer RJ. Esophageal cancer. N Engl J Med 2003;349(23): 2241–52.

24. Lepage C, Rachet B, Jooste V, et al. Continuing rapid increase in esophageal adenocarcinoma in England and Wales. Am J Gastroenterol 2008;103(11): 2694–9.

25. Pohl H, Welch HG. The role of overdiagnosis and reclassification in the marked increase of esophageal adenocarcinoma incidence. J Natl Cancer Inst 2005; 97(2):142–6.

26. De Stefani E, Barrios E, Fierro L. Black (air-cured) and blond (flue-cured) tobacco and cancer risk. III: Oesophageal cancer. Eur J Cancer 1993;29A(5):763–6.

27. Gammon MD, Schoenberg JB, Ahsan H, et al. Tobacco, alcohol, and socioeconomic status and adenocarcinomas of the esophagus and gastric cardia. J Natl Cancer Inst 1997;89(17):1277–84.

28. Lee CH, Wu DC, Lee JM, et al. Carcinogenetic impact of alcohol intake on squamous cell carcinoma risk of the oesophagus in relation to tobacco smoking. Eur J Cancer 2007;43(7):1188–99.

29. Polednak AP. Trends in survival for both histologic types of esophageal cancer in US surveillance, epidemiology and end results areas. Int J Cancer 2003;105(1): 98–100.

30. Ahsan H, Neugut AI. Radiation therapy for breast cancer and increased risk for esophageal carcinoma. Ann Intern Med 1998;128(2):114–7.

31. Brown LM, Hoover R, Silverman D, et al. Excess incidence of squamous cell esophageal cancer among US Black men: role of social class and other risk factors. Am J Epidemiol 2001;153(2):114–22.

32. Abnet CC, Lai B, Qiao YL, et al. Zinc concentration in esophageal biopsy specimens measured by x-ray fluorescence and esophageal cancer risk. J Natl Cancer Inst 2005;97(4):301–6.

33. Abnet CC, Qiao YL, Mark SD, et al. Prospective study of tooth loss and incident esophageal and gastric cancers in China. Cancer Causes Control 2001;12(9): 847–54.

34. Taylor PR, Qiao YL, Abnet CC, et al. Prospective study of serum vitamin E levels and esophageal and gastric cancers. J Natl Cancer Inst 2003;95(18):1414–6.

35. Risk JM, Mills HS, Garde J, et al. The tylosis esophageal cancer (TOC) locus: more than just a familial cancer gene. Dis Esophagus 1999;12(3):173–6.

36. Blaydon DC, Etheridge SL, Risk JM, et al. RHBDF2 mutations are associated with tylosis, a familial esophageal cancer syndrome. Am J Hum Genet 2012;90(2): 340–6.
37. Reid BJ, Li X, Galipeau PC, et al. Barrett's oesophagus and oesophageal adenocarcinoma: time for a new synthesis. Nat Rev Cancer 2010;10(2):87–101.
38. Engel LS, Chow WH, Vaughan TL, et al. Population attributable risks of esophageal and gastric cancers. J Natl Cancer Inst 2003;95(18):1404–13.
39. Pennathur A, Landreneau RJ, Luketich JD. Surgical aspects of the patient with high-grade dysplasia. Semin Thorac Cardiovasc Surg 2005;17(4):326–32.
40. Bornschein J, Selgrad M, Warnecke M, et al. H. pylori infection is a key risk factor for proximal gastric cancer. Dig Dis Sci 2010;55(11):3124–31.
41. Wu MS, Shun CT, Wu CC, et al. Epstein-Barr virus-associated gastric carcinomas: relation to H. pylori infection and genetic alterations. Gastroenterology 2000; 118(6):1031–8.
42. Wang HH, Wu MS, Shun CT, et al. Lymphoepithelioma-like carcinoma of the stomach: a subset of gastric carcinoma with distinct clinicopathological features and high prevalence of Epstein-Barr virus infection. Hepatogastroenterology 1999; 46(26):1214–9.
43. Oliveira C, Pinheiro H, Figueiredo J, et al. Familial gastric cancer: genetic susceptibility, pathology, and implications for management. Lancet Oncol 2015;16(2): e60–70.
44. Lunet N, Valbuena C, Vieira AL, et al. Fruit and vegetable consumption and gastric cancer by location and histological type: case-control and meta-analysis. Eur J Cancer Prev 2007;16(4):312–27.
45. Ladeiras-Lopes R, Pereira AK, Nogueira A, et al. Smoking and gastric cancer: systematic review and meta-analysis of cohort studies. Cancer Causes Control 2008;19(7):689–701.
46. Yang P, Zhou Y, Chen B, et al. Overweight, obesity and gastric cancer risk: results from a meta-analysis of cohort studies. Eur J Cancer 2009;45(16):2867–73.
47. Bass AJ, Watanabe H, Mermel CH, et al. SOX2 is an amplified lineage-survival oncogene in lung and esophageal squamous cell carcinomas. Nat Genet 2009;41(11):1238–42.
48. Lawrence MS, Stojanov P, Polak P, et al. Mutational heterogeneity in cancer and the search for new cancer-associated genes. Nature 2013;499(7457):214–8.
49. Dhupar R, Van Der Kraak L, Pennathur A, et al. Targeting immune checkpoints in esophageal cancer: a high mutational load tumor. Ann Thorac Surg 2017;103(4): 1340–9.
50. Lee RC, Feinbaum RL, Ambros V. The C. elegans heterochronic gene lin-4 encodes small RNAs with antisense complementarity to lin-14. Cell 1993;75(5): 843–54.
51. Esquela-Kerscher A, Slack FJ. Oncomirs - microRNAs with a role in cancer. Nat Rev Cancer 2006;6(4):259–69.
52. Rabinovitch PS, Longton G, Blount PL, et al. Predictors of progression in Barrett's esophagus III: baseline flow cytometric variables. Am J Gastroenterol 2001; 96(11):3071–83.
53. Morales CP, Souza RF, Spechler SJ. Hallmarks of cancer progression in Barrett's oesophagus. Lancet 2002;360(9345):1587–9.
54. Feber A, Xi L, Pennathur A, et al. MicroRNA prognostic signature for nodal metastases and survival in esophageal adenocarcinoma. Ann Thorac Surg 2011;91(5): 1523–30.

55. Quackenbush J. Microarray analysis and tumor classification. N Engl J Med 2006;354(23):2463–72.
56. Shimada Y, Sato F, Shimizu K, et al. cDNA microarray analysis of esophageal cancer: discoveries and prospects. Gen Thorac Cardiovasc Surg 2009;57(7): 347–56.
57. Hu N, Wang C, Su H, et al. High frequency of CDKN2A alterations in esophageal squamous cell carcinoma from a high-risk Chinese population. Genes Chromosomes Cancer 2004;39(3):205–16.
58. National Center for Biotechnology Information. Available at: http://www.ncbi.nlm. nih.gov/gene/1029#reference-sequences. Accessed February 20, 2019.
59. Pennathur A, Farkas A, Krasinskas AM, et al. Esophagectomy for T1 esophageal cancer: outcomes in 100 patients and implications for endoscopic therapy. Ann Thorac Surg 2009;87(4):1048–54 [discussion: 1054–5].
60. Luketich JD, Schauer P, Landreneau R, et al. Minimally invasive surgical staging is superior to endoscopic ultrasound in detecting lymph node metastases in esophageal cancer. J Thorac Cardiovasc Surg 1997;114(5):817–21 [discussion: 821–3].
61. Kaushik N, Khalid A, Brody D, et al. Endoscopic ultrasound compared with laparoscopy for staging esophageal cancer. Ann Thorac Surg 2007;83(6):2000–2.
62. Mehta K, Bianco V, Awais O, et al. Minimally invasive staging of esophageal cancer. Ann Cardiothorac Surg 2017;6(2):110–8.
63. Xi L, Luketich JD, Raja S, et al. Molecular staging of lymph nodes from patients with esophageal adenocarcinoma. Clin Cancer Res 2005;11(3):1099–109.
64. Izbicki JR, Hosch SB, Pichlmeier U, et al. Prognostic value of immunohistochemically identifiable tumor cells in lymph nodes of patients with completely resected esophageal cancer. N Engl J Med 1997;337(17):1188–94.
65. Egyud MR, Tejani MA, Pennathur A, et al. Detection of circulating tumor DNA in plasma: a potential biomarker for esophageal adenocarcinoma. Ann Thorac Surg 2019. In press.

Multidisciplinary Therapy of Esophageal Cancer

Matthew R. Egyud, MD[a], Jennifer F. Tseng, MD, MPH[b],*, Kei Suzuki, MD[c]

KEYWORDS

- Esophageal cancer • Gastroesophageal junction tumor • Adenocarcinoma
- Squamous cell carcinoma • Multimodality therapy

KEY POINTS

- Multimodality therapy is the standard of care for locoregional esophageal cancers (greater than clinical T3 or N+), including Siewert type 1 and 2 gastroesophageal junction tumors.
- Induction regimen, chemotherapy only or chemoradiation, is an area of controversy and often institution-specific as neither has shown to be superior.
- Response to induction therapy has consistently shown to be an important prognostic marker.
- For esophageal squamous cell carcinoma, it may be acceptable to observe clinical complete responders after chemoradiotherapy and perform salvage esophagectomy for recurrent disease.
- Clinical T2N0 esophageal cancer presents a unique challenge given its inaccuracy in clinical staging. As such, management of this particular subset is controversial.

INTRODUCTION

Esophageal cancer is among the top 15 most commonly diagnosed cancers in the United States, and remains particularly lethal.[1] The primary management of esophageal and gastroesophageal junction (GEJ) cancer is variable depending on the underlying histology and disease stage. Esophageal squamous cell carcinoma (SCC) typically occurs in the proximal two-thirds of the esophagus and is primarily treated with chemoradiotherapy (CRT) with or without surgery. Adenocarcinoma (AC), including GEJ tumors, is generally treated with induction therapy and surgical resection, although controversy exits on the optimal induction regimen. Herein we review

Disclosures: The authors have nothing to disclose.
[a] Department of Surgery, Boston University School of Medicine, 88 East Newton Street, Collamore C-500, Boston, MA 02118, USA; [b] Department of Surgery, Boston University School of Medicine, Boston Medical Center, 88 East Newton Street, Collamore C-500, Boston, MA 02118, USA; [c] Department of Surgery, Boston University School of Medicine, Boston Medical Center, 88 East Newton Street, Robinson 7280, Boston, MA 02118, USA
* Corresponding author.
E-mail address: Jennifer.Tseng@bmc.org

the role of induction therapy, including chemotherapy and CRT, for loco-regionally advanced esophageal cancers.

ROLE OF INDUCTION THERAPY IN LOCO-REGIONALLY ADVANCED ESOPHAGEAL CANCER

When esophageal cancer invades through the muscularis propria and into the adventitia on endoscopic ultrasound (clinical T3) or has suspicious/biopsy-proven lymph node (N+), induction therapy is accepted as the current initial standard of care for both AC and SCC. Depth of invasion can be visualized using endoscopic ultrasound, which delineates layers of the esophagus with adequate resolution to permit assessment of clinical T stage (**Fig. 1**). Findings from main studies investigating the role of induction therapy in patients with resectable esophageal cancer are summarized in **Table 1**.

Induction Chemotherapy Versus Surgery Alone

We start with the question: *is preoperative chemotherapy efficacious for patients with surgically resectable esophageal cancer?* The UK Medical Research Council esophageal cancer trial (OEO2), published in 2009, compared induction chemotherapy followed by surgery versus surgery alone for patients with intrathoracic esophageal cancer (SCC, AC, or undifferentiated cancer), who were deemed resectable (staging not provided).[2–5] In total, 802 patients were recruited; 400 for induction chemotherapy with 2 cycles of cisplatin and fluorouracil and 402 for surgery alone. Patients undergoing induction had smaller-volume tumors ($P = .0001$) and had fewer involved nodes (58% vs 69%, $P = .009$). R0 resection rate was low overall but higher in the induction group (60%) compared with surgery-alone group (54%; $P<.0001$). Most importantly, survival data showed improved overall survival (OS) after induction therapy (512 days vs 405 days, $P = .004$). Disease-free survival (DFS) was also improved in the induction group ($P = .0014$). Patients generally tolerated induction well, and 83% demonstrated similar or improved World Health Organization (WHO) performance status after therapy. The study demonstrated the efficacy of preoperative chemotherapy in improving OS and DFS, with more complete surgical resection and less invasive disease after induction therapy for patients with resectable

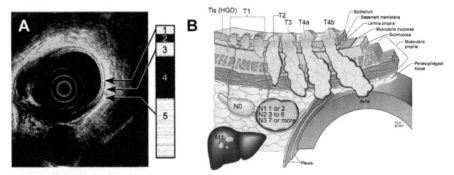

Fig. 1. (*A*) Endoscopic ultrasound image: first layer (hyperechoic, *white*) represents superficial mucosa (epithelium and lamina propria). Second layer (hypoechoic, *black*) represents deep mucosa (muscularis mucosa). Third layer (hyperechoic) represents submucosa. Fourth layer (hypoechoic) represents muscularis propria. Fifth layer (hyperechoic) represents periesophageal tissue. (*B*) Illustration demonstrates the depth of invasion. Tis: high-grade dysplasia. (Reprinted with permission, Cleveland Clinic Center for Medical Art & Photography © 2007–2019. All Rights Reserved.)

Table 1
Studies comparing multimodality approach with surgery alone for esophageal cancer

Study	Tumor Location	Histo	Preop Stage	Comparison	No. Pts	Chemo Regimen	Radiation Dose	R0 Rate, %	cPR Rate, %	Survival
OE02, *Lancet* 2002	Eso	AC, SCC, undiff	NR	Surgery	402	None	None	54	NR	Median OS 405 d
				Induction chemo + surgery	400	Cisplatin + fluorouracil		60		Median OS 512
Cunningham et al,[7] 2006 *N Engl J Med* (MAGIC)	Distal eso, GEJ, stomach	AC	Stage II-III	Surgery	253	None	None	70	NR	5-y OS 23%
				Surgery w/periop chemo	250	Epirubicin + cisplatin + fluorourcil		79		5-y OS 36%
Ychou et al,[8] 2011 *J Clin Oncol* (FNCLCC)	Distal eso, GEJ, stomach	AC	Any curative by resection	Surgery	111	None	None	74	NR	5-y OS 24%
				Surgery w/periop chemo	113	Cisplatin + fluorouracil		87		5-y OS 38%
Al-Batran et al,[9] 2016 *Lancet Oncol* (FLOT4)	GEJ, stomach	AC	>cT2, N+	Surgery w/periop chemo	152	Epirubicin + cisplatin + capecitabine/fluorouracil	None	74	6	N
					148	Fluorouracil + leucovorin + oxaliplatin + docetaxel		85	16	
van Hagen et al,[10] 2012 *N Engl J Med* (CROSS)	Eso, GEJ	AC, SCC, undiff	cT1N1, cT2-3N0-1	Surgery	188	None	None	69	NA	Median OS 24 mo
				Induction CRT + surgery	178	Carboplatin + paclitaxel	41.4 Gy	92	29% (23% AC) (49% SCC)	Median OS 49 mo

(continued on next page)

Table 1
(continued)

Study	Tumor Location	Histo	Preop Stage	Comparison	No. Pts	Chemo Regimen	Radiation Dose	R0 Rate, %	cPR Rate, %	Survival
Walsh et al,[12] 1996 *N Engl J Med*	Eso	AC	Any curative by resection	Surgery	55	None	None	NR	NA	3-y OS 6%
				Induction CRT + surgery	58	Fluorouracil + cisplatin	40 Gy	NR	25	3-y OS 32%
Tepper et al,[13] 2008 *J Clin Oncol* (CALGB 9781)	Eso	AC, SCC	Stage II-IVA	Surgery	26	None	None	NR	NR	Median OS 1.8 y 5-y OS 16%
				Induction CRT + surgery	30	Fluorouracil + cisplatin	50.5 Gy	NR	40	Median OS 4.5 y 5-y OS 39%
Klevebro et al,[14] 2016 *Ann Oncol* (NeoRes)	Eso, GEJ	AC, SCC	cT1-3 any N (no cT1N0)	Induction chemo + surgery	91	Cisplatin + fluorouracil	None	74	7% (AC) 16% (SCC)	3-y OS 49%
				Induction CRT + surgery	90	Cisplatin + fluorouracil	40 Gy	87	22% (AC) 42% (SCC)	3-y OS 47%
Burmeister et al,[15] 2011 *Eur J Cancer*	Eso, GEJ	AC	cT2-3, N0-1	Induction chemo + surgery	36	Cisplatin + fluorouracil	None	81	0	3-y OS 49% 5-y OS 36%
				Induction CRT + surgery	39	Cisplatin + fluorouracil	35 Gy	85	13	3-y OS 52% 5-y OS 45%

Study	Location	Histo	Stage	Treatment	Pts	Chemo	Radiation			Outcome
Stahl et al,[16] 2009 *J Clin Oncol* (POET)	Eso, GEJ	AC	cT3-4, Nx, M0	Induction chemo + surgery	59	Cisplatin, fluorouracil, leucovorin	None	70	2	3-y OS 26% 5-y OS 24%
				Induction CRT + surgery	60	Cisplatin, fluorouracil, leucovorin	30 Gy	72	16	3-y OS 47.7% 5-y OS 40%
Spicer et al,[17] 2016 *Ann Thorac Surg*	Eso, GEJ	AC	cT3N1M0	Induction chemo + surgery	114	Fluoropyrimidine + platinum-based vs taxane	None	87	7	Median OS 31 mo
				Induction CRT + surgery	100	Fluoropyrimidine + platinum-based vs taxane	50.4 Gy	99	17	Median OS 39 mo

Abbreviations: AC, adenocarcinoma; cPR, complete pathologic response; chemo, chemotherapy; CRT, chemoradiotherapy; Eso, esophagus; GEJ, gastroesophageal junction; Gy, Gray units of ionizing radiation; Histo, histology; NA, not applicable; NR, not reported; OS, overall survival; periop, perioperative; Pts, patients; SCC, squamous cell carcinoma; Undiff, undifferentiated cancer.

esophageal SCC or AC. This study established the efficacy of preoperative cisplatin/ fluorouracil as the standard of care for patients with esophageal cancer. Allum and colleagues[6] reviewed these results after a mean follow-up of 6 years of patients in the original trial. This confirmed the findings from the original study, with patients receiving induction chemotherapy experiencing prolonged DFS ($P = .003$) and OS ($P = .03$). This was demonstrated for both SCC and AC. Furthermore, patients with R0 resection showed a survival rate of 42.2% (median 2.1 years) versus R1 (18%, 1.1 years) and R2 (8.6%, 9 months).

Perioperative Chemotherapy Versus Surgery

Perioperative chemotherapy, defined as neoadjuvant plus postoperative therapy, improves survival in patients with esophageal cancer. We review here 3 major studies investigating the efficacy of perioperative chemotherapy for surgically resectable esophageal/GEJ cancers.

Medical Research Council adjuvant gastric infusional chemotherapy trial

The Medical Research Council adjuvant gastric infusional chemotherapy (MAGIC) trial assessed the addition of perioperative epirubicin, cisplatin, and fluorouracil (ECF) to surgical therapy for resectable AC of the stomach, GEJ, or lower esophagus.[7] In this study, 250 patients were recruited to perioperative chemotherapy and surgery versus 253 patients to surgery alone. Patients with histologically proven, surgically resectable stage II or higher distal esophageal/GEJ/gastric AC were included. In the perioperative chemotherapy group, 250 patients received 3 cycles each of both neoadjuvant and adjuvant chemotherapy, with surgery 3 to 6 weeks after completion of the third cycle of induction therapy, and resumption of chemotherapy 6 to 12 weeks postoperatively. Groups were similar with respect to age, sex, WHO performance status, location of tumor, and maximum tumor diameter. Notably, most tumors (74% perioperative therapy vs 68.4% surgery alone) were primary gastric AC. Of patients undergoing surgery, curative resection occurred in 79% of patients with perioperative therapy versus 70% with surgery-only patients. Tumors in perioperative chemotherapy patients had smaller diameters than surgery-only patients (median 3 cm vs 5 cm, $P<.001$), plus more patients were T1 and T2 (51.7% perioperative chemotherapy vs 36.8% surgery only, $P = .0002$). Perioperative chemotherapy improved DFS and OS ($P<.0001$), with 5-year OS of 36% in perioperative chemotherapy versus 23% in surgery alone.

Although fewer than 50% of study subjects completed the full course of chemotherapy, this study demonstrated the efficacy of perioperative chemotherapy in improving OS and DFS for patients with resectable AC of the stomach, GEJ, or distal esophagus. Based on this trial, perioperative ECF became the standard of care in the Western countries (Western Europe and the United States) for resectable esophagogastric cancers.

Fédération National des Centers de Luttre contre le Cancer

The Fédération National des Centers de Luttre contre le Cancer (FNCLCC) trial assessed the addition of perioperative fluorouracil plus cisplatin to surgical resection for gastroesophageal AC.[8] Patients with biopsy-proven, surgically resectable distal third esophageal, GEJ, or gastric AC were included. In total, 224 patients were recruited, with 113 randomized to perioperative chemotherapy and 111 to surgery alone. Chemotherapy patients underwent 2 to 3 cycles of neoadjuvant cisplatin + fluorouracil, followed by surgery 4 to 6 weeks after, and 3 to 4 cycles of adjuvant therapy. Surgery in both groups consisted of resection of the tumor to adequate margins with extended lymphadenectomy, with the approach being surgeon-dependent. Approximately 75% of patients in each group had distal esophageal/GEJ tumors. OS was improved for patients undergoing perioperative chemotherapy over surgery alone (P = .02). Patients undergoing perioperative chemotherapy alone had a higher rate of DFS (38% vs 19%, P = .01) and R0 resection rate (87% vs 74%, P = .004). Thirty-eight percent of patients undergoing perioperative chemotherapy experienced grade 3 to 4 toxicity. The 5-year OS benefit of 14% from perioperative chemotherapy came at the cost of a 73% rate of grade 3 to 4 toxicity, which was felt to be a limitation for this regimen.

Fluorouracil, leucovorin, oxaliplatin, and docetaxel

The Fluorouracil, Leucovorin, Oxaliplatin, and Docetaxel (FLOT4) study was a randomized study comparing 2 perioperative chemotherapy regimens.[9] Eligibility criteria included histologically confirmed gastric or GEJ AC, clinical stage T2 or higher or node positive by cross-sectional imaging or endoscopic ultrasound. Patients were randomized to perioperative epirubicin/cisplatin/capecitabine (ECX) or ECF given in 3 neoadjuvant and 3 adjuvant fractions, or fluorouracil/leucovorin/oxaliplatin/docetaxel (FLOT) given in 4 neoadjuvant and 4 adjuvant fractions. After preoperative chemotherapy, restaging was completed by computed tomography (CT) or MRI and endoscopy before surgical resection. Surgery was performed 3 weeks after the final cycle of preoperative chemotherapy. Type of surgical resection was dictated by location of the primary tumor.

In total, 300 patients were randomized; 152 to ECF/ECX and 148 to FLOT. Groups were similar with respect to age, sex, Eastern Cooperative Oncology Group (ECOG) performance status, tumor/node stage, and Lauren classification. There was a difference between groups based on primary tumor location as the FLOT group were more likely to have gastric cancer (52% vs 43%) and hence underwent a gastrectomy (X vs Y). More patients in the FLOT group underwent surgical resection as compared with ECF/ECX (119%, 93% vs 111%, 81%), with the most common reasons for no resection being progression of disease/death (11 patients) or metastatic disease on staging laparoscopy (16 patients). Patients undergoing FLOT had a significantly higher rate of pathologic complete response (pCR) compared with ECF/ECX (16% vs 6%, P = .02), and a higher rate of complete response/subtotal regression (37% vs 23%, P = .02). Tumor regression grading was compared relative to preoperative Lauren classification. Patients with intestinal-type tumors showed higher rates of TRG1a/b than diffuse gastric-type tumors. Response rates were not statistically significant between groups, but intestinal-type tumors treated with FLOT had a trend toward improved TRG1a response rate (20% vs 10%, P = .07). Rates of all serious adverse events and mortality were similar between groups.

The study demonstrated that FLOT regimen compared with ECF/ECX provided an increased chance of pCR and higher rate of surgical resection. Based on this study, FLOT warrants consideration as a new perioperative regimen in patients with resectable GEJ AC.

Induction Chemoradiotherapy Versus Surgery Alone

If induction chemotherapy confers a survival benefit in patients with surgically resectable esophageal cancer, *would induction chemoradiotherapy be efficacious compared with surgical resection alone?* In this section, we review studies that investigate the role of induction CRT in comparison with surgical resection alone.

ChemoRadiotherapy for oesophageal cancer followed by surgery study

The ChemoRadiotherapy for Oesophageal Cancer Followed by Surgery Study (CROSS) trial was a randomized trial comparing induction CRT followed by surgery versus surgery alone in patients with esophageal or GEJ tumors.[10,11] Patients with potentially curable, histologically confirmed AC, SCC, or undifferentiated carcinoma were enrolled; patients with cT1N1 or T2-3N0-1 without metastasis, plus WHO performance status 0 to 2 were eligible. Those randomized to CRT underwent treatment with carboplatin and paclitaxel with concomitant radiotherapy (41.4 Gy over 23 fractions) before surgery, whereas surgery-only patients underwent upfront surgical resection with a transthoracic esophagectomy. No postoperative therapy was administered. In total, 366 patients were included in the final analysis; 178 randomized to induction CRT whereas 188 were randomized to surgery alone. Groups were similar with respect to age, sex, tumor type, tumor location, and T and N stage. There were no significant differences in the rate of postoperative complications between the 2 groups. Under an intent-to-treat analysis, median OS in the CRT group was 49.4 months versus 24.0 months in the surgery-only group (P = .003). Rates of R0 resection were significantly different; 92% (n = 148) of CRT patients versus 69% (n = 111) of surgery-only patients (P<.001). pCR was reported in 49% (n = 47) of the CRT group; 23% AC (n = 28) versus 49% SCC (n = 18), although this histologic difference was not a prognostic factor for OS. Fewer patients undergoing CRT had positive lymph nodes (31%, n = 50) compared with surgery alone (n = 120, 75%) (P<.001).

The study demonstrated improved OS with induction CRT compared with surgery alone without increased perioperative morbidity or mortality. On long-term follow-up of patients in the CROSS trial, Shapiro and colleagues[11] corroborated these findings, noting improved median OS for CRT over surgery alone in both AC and SCC. Although critics argue against the inclusion of both AC and SCC in the study (larger effects seen in SCC), this study established induction CRT as the standard of care for esophageal and GEJ cancers.

Additional studies

Other studies have also investigated the role of the multimodality approach. Walsh and colleagues,[12] in their 1995 study, investigated the role of induction CRT consisting of 2 cycles of fluorouracil and cisplatin and 40 Gy followed by surgical resection and compared the outcome with surgical resection alone. Their study included only esophageal AC. The study conferred a survival benefit to the multimodality approach, with a significant difference in 3-year OS (32% for multimodality vs 6% for surgery alone, P = .01). This study occurred before many of the modern modifications to chemotherapy and administration of radiotherapy. CALGB 9781 was a study comparing a trimodality approach with surgery alone for nonmetastatic esophageal cancer. The study included both AC and SCC.[13] The trimodality regimen consisted of induction fluorouracil/cisplatin and 50.5 Gy followed by surgery versus surgical resection alone. Although this randomized trial was closed because of poor accrual (56 patients), it did demonstrate a survival benefit for the multimodality group: median survival of 4.5 versus 1.8 years (P = .002) and 5-year OS of 39% vs 16%.

Induction Chemotherapy Versus Induction Chemoradiotherapy

The previously discussed studies demonstrated the efficacy of the multimodality approach to loco-regionally advanced esophageal cancer. The exact regimen, however, has been an area of debate. As such, the multimodality treatment is oftentimes institution-specific. *What is the ideal induction therapy: chemotherapy or chemoradiation?* In this section, we review the studies comparing induction chemotherapy vs chemoradiotherapy.

Neoadjuvant chemotherapy versus radiochemotherapy for cancer of the esophagus or cardia (NeoRes)

The NeoRes trial was a randomized trial comparing induction chemotherapy versus induction CRT.[14] Patients with SCC or AC, including GEJ tumors, eligible for surgical resection (T1-3, any N, except T1N0) were included. Chemotherapy included 3 cycles of cisplatin and fluorouracil. Patients randomized to receive CRT also received 40 Gy over 20 fractions with cycles 2 to 3. Patients then underwent appropriate resection; operation type was based on the tumor location.

In total, 181 patients were randomized; 91 underwent neoadjuvant chemotherapy and 90 underwent CRT: both groups were similar with respect to age, tumor type/location stage, and surgical approach. Each group had 78 patients subsequently undergoing esophagectomy. Rate of postoperative complications were similar between both groups, although severity was increased with addition of radiotherapy. Patients with SCC had higher rates of resection in the CRT group compared with chemotherapy only (n = 24, 96% vs n = 19, 75%, P = .04) whereas AC had similar rates of resection. Among surgical patients, rates of pCR (28% vs 9%, P = .002) and R0 resection (87% vs 74%, P = .04) were higher in the CRT group and these patients had lower rates of lymph node metastasis (35% vs 62%, P = .001). For survival, 3-year OS was similar between groups, before and after stratification by histologic subtype. However, there was a trend toward improved survival with radiotherapy in SCC, and worse survival with radiotherapy in AC. In this study, pCR was not a marker for survival.

The study demonstrated that induction CRT increases the rate of pCR, R0 resection, and negative nodes, but does not confer a survival advantage. CRT did, however, demonstrate a trend toward improving survival in SCC.

Burmeister and colleagues 2011: chemoradiation versus chemotherapy

Burmeister and colleagues[15] set out to assess the benefit of induction chemotherapy alone versus CRT in esophageal AC. Patients with esophageal and GEJ AC were included if they were surgical candidates and had not received any prior chemotherapy or radiation. Patients were randomized into either chemotherapy with 2 cycles of cisplatin and fluorouracil, or CRT with the same chemotherapy regimen plus 35 Gy radiotherapy over 15 fractions. If patients were without systemic disease at restaging, they underwent esophagectomy. In total, 75 patients were randomized: 36 patients underwent chemotherapy and 39 underwent CRT. Groups were similar with regard to age, ECOG status, stage, and surgical approach. Of the chemotherapy-only patients, 21 completed therapy per protocol, and 33 underwent surgery, whereas in CRT, 23 completed chemotherapy and 34 completed radiotherapy, and 33 underwent surgery. Rates and type of toxicity from therapy and surgical complications were similar between both groups, although CRT trended toward significance for wound infections. Rate of R0 resection was higher in CRT versus chemotherapy only (100% vs 86%, P = .04). DFS and OS were similar between both groups.

The study demonstrated that adding concurrent radiotherapy to preoperative chemotherapy did not increase morbidity or mortality, and did increase R0 resection rates, but not survival.

PreOperative therapy in esophagogastric adenocarcinoma trial

Stahl and colleagues[16] performed a randomized controlled trial comparing induction chemotherapy with CRT in GEJ AC. Patients were included if they had T3 or T4 disease, no prior treatment, and were surgical candidates. Patients were prospectively randomized to receive chemotherapy with cisplatin, fluorouracil, and leucovorin in 2.5 cycles, or CRT with the same chemotherapy regimen in 2 cycles followed by 3 subsequent weeks of cisplatin and etoposide plus concurrent 30 Gy radiation. Patients then underwent esophagectomy based on the surgeon's preference. In total, 119 patients were randomized: 59 patients received chemotherapy with 52 subsequently undergoing surgery, whereas 60 patients received CRT and 49 patients subsequently underwent surgery. Patients undergoing CRT were statistically older, but groups were otherwise similar. Rates of toxicity from therapy were similar between both groups. The main reasons for exclusion from surgery were because of disease progression or decline in performance status. Rates of R0 resection were similar, although pCR was higher in the CRT group ($P = .03$). CRT was associated with a trend toward improved OS ($P = .07$) at 3 years and less tumor progression on therapy ($P = .06$) Subanalysis of pathologic nodal status, irrespective of treatment arm, noted an increased 3-year survival for negative nodes (76.5% vs 59.0%, respectively, $P<.001$). This remained true when further divided by treatment arm.

The study demonstrated that adding concurrent radiotherapy to preoperative chemotherapy improved DFS and OS without increase in morbidity, although they note that their sample size limited their ability to provide statistical significance for this finding. Initial results were published in 2009, with updated results published in 2017, as the initial trial did not meet its primary endpoint of survival at 3 years. At this reanalysis, OS still trended toward significance in favor of CRT ($P = .055$), and local progression-free survival remained statistically significant ($P = .01$).

Spicer and colleagues 2016: chemoradiation versus chemotherapy before esophagectomy

Spicer and colleagues[17] reviewed 3 prospective databases of patients undergoing induction chemotherapy versus CRT for esophageal and GEJ AC. Included patients had cT3N1 disease, and underwent induction chemotherapy versus CRT, followed by en bloc esophagectomy. Patients underwent varying cycles of chemotherapy with a fluoropyrimidine and platinum-based agent versus taxane. Patients undergoing CRT had the same chemotherapy plus 50.4 Gy of radiation. Surgical resection, via en bloc esophagectomy with D2 and mediastinal lymphadenectomy, plus possible cervical lymphadenectomy based on tumor location, occurred 4 to 6 weeks after therapy. Across 3 databases, 214 patients were included. There were no significant differences between the 2 groups with respect to demographics, preoperative comorbidities, and tumor differentiation. Of the 3 databases, 1 site used only CRT, a second used only chemotherapy, and a third used both modalities. Surgical approaches differed among institutions in terms of fields of lymphadenectomy, thus there were significant differences in the number of patients undergoing 3-field esophagectomy after chemotherapy (39.8%) versus CRT (7%). This led to differences in the rate of cervical anastomoses. Groups were similar in rates of R0 resection. Morbidity and mortality rates were similar between groups, including anastomotic leaks (CRT 15% vs chemo alone 11.6%, $P = .54$). There were no significant differences in OS or DFS, although CRT trended toward improved DFS (26.4 months vs 16.0 months, $P = .135$). Site of recurrence was similar between cohorts. Field of resection and number of positive nodes both independently correlated with poor outcomes.

This review demonstrated that there is no OS or DFS difference between induction CRT and chemotherapy before esophagectomy, although there is a trend to improved DFS with CRT. Number of fields of lymphadenectomy were an independent predictor of worse outcomes. There were interinstitutional treatment differences in surgical approach that must also be considered. Thus, they concluded both treatment modalities are acceptable, so long as en bloc esophagectomy follows neoadjuvant therapy.

Sjoquist and colleagues 2011: meta-analysis of neoadjuvant chemotherapy versus chemoradiotherapy

Sjoquist and colleagues[18] had previously performed a meta-analysis demonstrating a survival benefit using induction therapy (chemotherapy or CRT) before esophagectomy (ref), and updated this meta-analysis in 2011. A total of 24 randomized controlled trials with intention-to-treat met inclusion criteria and were included for analysis. Twelve studies compared CRT with surgery, 9 compared chemotherapy with surgery, 2 compared induction CRT and chemotherapy, and 1 compared all: CRT, chemotherapy, and radiotherapy with surgery. In all, 4188 patients were included across all trials. Induction CRT, compared with surgery alone, showed a statistically significant survival benefit of 8.7% over 2 years ($P<.0001$), both for SCC ($P = .004$) and AC ($P = .02$). Induction chemotherapy, compared with surgery alone, showed a 2-year 5.1% survival benefit ($P = .005$). This benefit remained statistically significant for AC only ($P = .01$). Induction CRT, compared with induction chemotherapy, showed no survival benefit, although both of these trials were underpowered due to early closure. The review concluded that there is a survival advantage for induction therapy (both CRT and chemotherapy) over surgical monotherapy, and that this benefit applies to both SCC and AC. Induction CRT, once again, did not show any added benefit when compared with induction chemotherapy.

Open trials

Based on these studies, the question of induction chemotherapy versus CRT still remains unanswered. There are a couple important ongoing trials that may shed some light. The NEOadjuvant Trial in Adenocarcinoma of the esophagus and oesophago-Gastric Junction International Study (Neo-AEGIS) is a randomized trial comparing the 2 established regimens for esophageal and GEJ tumors: perioperative chemo per MAGIC regimen versus the induction CRT per CROSS regimen.[19] The Trial of Preoperative therapy for Gastric and Esophagogastric junction AdenocaRcinoma (TOP-GEAR) trial is another randomized phase III comparison of perioperative chemotherapy per MAGIC regimen versus the same regimen with the addition of 45 Gy of induction radiation.[20] The Perioperative Chemotherapy Compared to Neoadjuvant Chemoradiation in Patients with Adenocarcinoma of the Esophagus (ESOPEC) trial is a prospective trial comparing a perioperative chemotherapy regimen per the FLOT protocol (fluorouracil, leucovorin, oxaliplatin, and docetaxel) with induction CRT per the CROSS protocol. Patients with resectable AC of the esophagus, including Siewert 1 GEJ and some patients with Siewert 2 and 3 with evidence of esophageal infiltration will be included in the study.[21]

Squamous Cell Carcinoma

In the CROSS trial, analysis of pathology specimen revealed complete response in 29% of patients: 49% for SCC and 23% for AC. The high rate of pCR, especially in SCC, combined with the morbid nature of esophagectomy, has led some to consider a surveillance approach in treating patients with SCC. *What is the value of surgery in addition to CRT in patients with SCC?* In this section, we first review studies comparing CRT as the primary therapy versus trimodality approach (**Table 2**). We then review studies assessing the role of salvage esophagectomy.

Stahl and colleagues[22] compared CRT versus CRT plus surgery in locoregional esophageal SCC (cT3-4, N0-1, M0) in the upper/mid third thoracic esophagus. The study population is appropriately staged and homogeneous. In their study, 172 patients were randomized to trimodality therapy (chemotherapy followed by CRT with 40 Gy followed by surgery) or chemotherapy followed by definitive CRT, with at least

Table 2
Studies comparing chemoradiation with or without surgery for esophageal cancer

Study	Study Type	Histo	Preop Stage	Comparison	No. Pts	Chemo Regimen	Radiation Dose	R0 Rate, %	cPR Rate, %	Survival	Mortality, %	Main Conclusion
Stahl et al,[22] 2005 *J Clin Oncol*	Randomized	SCC	cT3-4, N0-1	CRT	86	Fluorouracil + leucovorin + etoposide + cisplatin	≥65 Gy	NA	NA	2-y OS 35%	3.5	Addition of surgery improves local control but not OS.
				CRT + surgery	86		40 Gy	82	35	2-y OS 40%	13	
Bedenne et al,[23] 2007 *J Clin Oncol* (FFCD 9102)	Randomized	AC & SCC	cT3N0-1	CRT	130	Fluorouracil + cisplatin	66 Gy	NR	NR	2-y OS 40%	1	Addition of surgery improves local control but not OS.
				CRT + surgery	129		46 Gy	75	23	2-y OS 34%	9	
Markar et al,[24] 2015 *J Clin Oncol* (SALV)	Retrospective	SCC, ACC, other	cI-IV	CRT + planed surgery	540	NR	Median 45 Gy	89	23	3-y OS 43%	11	Salvage esophagectomy results in acceptable outcome.
				CRT + salvage surgery	308		Median 50 Gy	87	22	3-y OS 40%	8	

Abbreviations: AC, adenocarcinoma; cPR, complete pathologic response; CRT, chemoradiotherapy; Eso, esophagus; Gy, Gray units of ionizing radiation; Histo, histology; NA, not applicable; NR, not reported; OS, overall survival; Pts, patients; SCC, squamous cell carcinoma.

65 Gy. The surgery arm had better local control, as evidenced by 2-year progression-free survival of 64% compared with 41% in the CRT arm (P = .003). However, this did not result in improved survival: 2-year OS was 40% for the surgery arm and 35% for CRT arm. In addition, treatment-related mortality was significantly higher in the surgery arm (13% vs 3.5%, P = .03). Another important finding from this study is that response to induction chemotherapy was an independent prognostic factor. Response was assessed by a combination of dysphagia improvement and measurements based on CT or barium esophagram. Subgroup analysis revealed that responders had significantly better prognosis, and that the addition of surgery in this particular group did not change outcome. On the other hand, in nonresponders, those who had complete resection showed improved survival compared with the nonsurgical group.

In the French study FFCD 9102, Bedenne and colleagues[23] randomized 259 patients with T3N0-1M0 esophageal cancer (both AC and SCC) to CRT only or CRT followed by surgery. Both groups received CRT consisting of fluorouracil/cisplatin and 46 Gy radiation. They were then randomized to undergo surgery or continue CRT. The study population was mainly SCC (89%). No difference in survival was observed: 2-year OS of 34% for the surgery arm versus 40% for CRT despite improved local control in the surgery arm. In a subgroup analysis of those who responded to induction chemotherapy, 3-year OS was similar in both groups.

Results of these 2 randomized trials indicate that for SCC, definitive CRT is an acceptable therapy, especially in those who show response to induction therapy and those who may not tolerate the rigors of esophagectomy. As such, additional predictive and prognostic markers as well as a better way to assess tumor response would move the field forward.

For those patients undergoing definitive CRT in whom disease recurs or is deemed persistent, salvage esophagectomy can be considered. The SALV trial assessed the impact of salvage esophagectomy after definitive CRT for esophageal cancers.[24] Data were collected retrospectively for patients undergoing planned surgery after induction CRT (n = 540) and patients undergoing salvage esophagectomy (n = 308), and further compared patients who benefited from salvage esophagectomy in the setting of persistent disease versus recurrent disease after definitive CRT. Both OS and DFS were similar for planned surgery and salvage surgery (3-year OS 43% vs 40%, P = .54; 3-year DFS 39% vs 33%, P = .23). When comparing persistent versus recurrent disease within the salvage group, 3-year OS was better in recurrent disease (56%) compared with persistent disease (41%, P = .046), with a similar trend seen in DFS (3-year DFS 52% for recurrent vs 37% for persistent, P = .095). The study demonstrates that salvage esophagectomy results in acceptable outcomes.

For patients who are deemed to have clinical complete response, the role of surgery also has been questioned. There is an ongoing trial in the Netherlands (the SANO trial) that is randomizing clinical complete responders to either surgery or surveillance.[25] Another important question in this subgroup is how to accurately deem someone a clinical complete responder. In the SANO trial, this is done by repeat endoscopy with bite-on-bite biopsy as well as endoscopic ultrasound and PET-CT.

The Metabolic Response Evaluation for Individualization of Neoadjuvant Chemotherapy in Oesophageal and Oesophagogastric Adenocarcinoma

As response to induction chemotherapy has shown prognostic value in many studies, another important question in the management of esophageal cancers is: *how can we assess response to induction therapy?* The Metabolic Response Evaluation for

Individualization of Neoadjuvant Chemotherapy in Oesophageal and Oesophagogastric Adenocarcinoma (MUNICON) trial was a phase II prospective trial assessing the utility of PET-CT early during induction chemotherapy for predicting metabolic response and survival.[26–28] Patients with stage cT3 or cT4 GEJ AC (Siewert 1 or 2) who were candidates for chemotherapy were included. All patients received a PET-CT within 1 week before initiation of chemotherapy, and patients without sufficient differences in standard uptake value (SUV) between the tumor and local normal tissue were excluded. All patients then underwent platinum and fluorouracil-based chemotherapy, and a repeat PET was performed after 14 days. Patients with decrease in SUV max of at least 35% were considered responders to chemotherapy and continued chemotherapy for up to 12 total weeks, whereas nonresponders (SUV max increase or decrease <35%) were stratified to undergoing surgery. All patients underwent 2 cycles of cisplatin or oxaliplatin with folinic acid, plus fluorouracil. Patients younger than 60 years who were otherwise fairly healthy were also given paclitaxel. Endoscopy and repeat CT staging were performed to evaluate for tumor progression. Surgery was scheduled within 2 weeks for nonresponders, and 4 weeks for responders based on the PET-CT. Patients with Siewert type 1 tumors then underwent abdominothoracic esophagectomy, whereas patients with Siewert type 2 tumors underwent transhiatal extended gastrectomy. In total, 119 consecutive patients were recruited with 8 subsequently excluded, and 54 of 110 surviving patients were deemed as responders. Responders versus nonresponders were similar with regard to age, sex, tumor location, T and N stage, and performance status. Responders, on pathologic examination, tended to have more poorly differentiated tumors with higher initial SUVs ($P = .018$). Among those undergoing surgery, 88 patients underwent R0 resection with the remaining 16 patients with R1 resections. Rate of R0 resection was increased in responders (96% vs 74%, $P = .002$). Rate of postoperative complications were similar between responders and nonresponders. Of the 50 responders, 29 showed a major histopathologic response (<10% remaining viable tumor) with 8 complete responders, and 21 with subtotal remission. Retroactive assessment of the SUV decrease did not show statistical significance between complete responders and subtotal responders. Median event-free survival was increased in responders (29.7 months vs 14.1 months, $P = .002$) as was median OS: 25.8 months in nonresponders and not reached in responders ($P = .015$). Responders with a major histopathologic response had improved OS ($P = .004$) and DFS ($P = .006$) compared with responders with subtotal remission on pathology. Metabolic responders without histologic response showed similar survival compared with nonresponders.

The study demonstrates that PET-CT early during induction chemotherapy can demonstrate early metabolic response correlating with major histologic responses, which carries a survival advantage for distal esophageal and GEJ AC. Incorporating this into an algorithm for treatment can allow patients with response to undergo their full course of chemotherapy, whereas those without response to avoid weeks of ineffective chemotherapy and potential loss of surgical candidacy via disease progression.

ROLE OF INDUCTION THERAPY IN EARLY-STAGE ESOPHAGEAL CANCER

For early-stage (stages I-II) esophageal cancers, the current gold standard of care is esophagectomy. However, there are studies that investigated the efficacy of multimodality therapy in this population. *Is there a role for multimodality approach in patients with early-stage esophageal cancer?* We review studies investigating this question (**Table 3**).

Table 3
Studies investigating role of induction therapy in early-stage esophageal cancer

Study	Study Type	Histo	Preop Stage	Comparison	No. Pts	R0 Rate, %	cPR Rate, %	Survival	Mortality, %
Mariette et al,[29] 2014 *J Clin Oncol* (FFC 9901)	Randomized	AC, SCC, other	cI–II	Surgery CRT + surgery	97 98	92 94	NA 36	3-y OS 53% 3-y OS 48%	1 7
Markar et al,[30] 2016 *Eur J Cancer*	Retrospective	NR	cT2N0	Surgery Induction therapy + surgery	152 148	92 93	NA 19	Median OS 43 mo Median OS 39 mo	7 9
Speicher et al,[31] 2014 *J Thorac Oncol*	Retrospective (NCDB)	NR	cT2N0	Surgery Induction therapy + surgery	871 688	91 96	NA 6	Median OS 41 mo Median OS 42 mo	4 3.5
Martin et al,[32] 2013 *Ann Thorac Surg*	Retrospective (SEER)	AC, SCC	cT2N0	Surgery Surgery + radiation	267 223	NR NR	NA NR	5-y OS 39% 5-y OS 42%	NR NR

Abbreviations: AC, adenocarcinoma; cPR, complete pathologic response; CRT, chemoradiotherapy; Eso, esophagus; Histo, histology; NCDB, national cancer database; NA, not applicable; NR, not reported; OS, overall survival; SCC, squamous cell carcinoma; SEER, surveillance, epidemiology, and end results.

In FFCD 9901, Mariette and colleagues[29] randomized 195 patients with stage I-II esophageal cancer to surgery alone (n = 97) or induction therapy (fluorouracil/cisplatin and 45 Gy radiation) followed by surgery (n = 98). Addition of induction therapy did not improve the R0 resection rate (94% for induction vs 92% for surgery, $P = .75$) or survival (3-year OS 48% for induction vs 53% for surgery, $P = .94$).

In a large retrospective review, Markar and colleagues[30] investigated 355 patients with cT2N0 esophageal cancer. Although the induction group had significantly more downstaging, no survival benefit was seen with the addition of the induction therapy. Of note, nearly 50% of patients had nodal disease on pathologic analysis.

In a review of the National Cancer Database in the Unites States, Speicher and colleagues[31] reported their findings from a review of more than 1500 patients staged cT2N0. Again, there was no survival benefit conferred with the addition of induction therapy (median OS 41 months for surgery alone vs 42 months for induction therapy, $P = .51$). Among those who underwent surgery as the primary therapy, 42% of patients were upstaged and 32% of patients were down-staged.

Another retrospective review of the SEER (Surveillance, Epidemiology, and End Results) database for cT2N0 patients comparing addition of radiation with surgery was performed by Martin and colleagues.[32] This review of 490 patients did not show any survival benefit with the addition of radiation.

The clinical dilemma in patients with cT2N0 esophageal cancer goes beyond the question of what the appropriate treatment is. The clinical staging in this subset is notorious for being imprecise: 27% to 56% of patients are understaged on pathologic analysis,[33] whereas 39% to 55% of patients are known to have lymph node involvement on resected specimen.[34,35]

For those who are understaged or are truly T2N0, it would make sense to proceed with surgical resection, as the addition of induction therapy has not shown any survival benefit. For those who are upstaged, multimodality therapy with induction therapy followed by surgical resection may make sense, but the barrier to accurate staging still exits. As such, this subgroup represents a clinical population in need of additional clinical or biologic markers to further delineate who should receive surgical resection versus who would benefit from induction therapy.

SUMMARY

Management of loco-regionally advanced esophageal cancers continues to present clinical challenges because of controversies in different areas. For those who are surgical candidates, the multimodality approach remains the standard of care. Studies such as OE02 and MAGIC set the standard by showing efficacy of neoadjuvant and perioperative chemotherapy compared with surgery alone, whereas studies such as the CROSS trial set the standard by demonstrating the efficacy of induction CRT. Although most agree on the efficacy of induction therapy, the exact regimen, whether to include radiation as part of induction, remains an area of controversy, as most studies comparing induction chemotherapy versus CRT have not shown a significant difference. As such, the exact treatment management/modality remains institution-specific.

Another area of controversy is the management of patients with SCC, partly because they tend to respond better to CRT. Salvage esophagectomy appears to have equal efficacy compared with planned resection. For those who show complete response, definitive CRT also may be an acceptable approach.

One area for improvement is the need for markers of response to induction therapy, especially because tumor response in many studies have shown prognostic significance. The MUNICON study showed evidence that PET-CT may be used in this fashion, whereas in an ongoing Dutch trial, a bite-on-bite biopsy is being used. There is also a need for marker in the cT2N0 population, as this subgroup is notorious for being imprecisely staged. Because this population could be treated with upfront surgery or multimodality approach, a marker to tailor treatment in this subgroup is an area of investigation.

REFERENCES

1. Cronin KA, Lake AJ, Scott S, et al. Annual report to the nation on the status of cancer, part I: national cancer statistics. Cancer 2018;124(13):2785–800.
2. Bosset JF, Mercier M, Triboulet JP, et al. Surgical resection with and without chemotherapy in oesophageal cancer. Lancet 2002;360(9340):1173–4 [author reply: 1175].
3. Chander S. Surgical resection with and without chemotherapy in oesophageal cancer. Lancet 2002;360(9340):1174 [author reply: 1175].
4. Maraveyas A, O'Boyle C, Cowen M. Surgical resection with and without chemotherapy in oesophageal cancer. Lancet 2002;360(9340):1174–5 [author reply: 1175].
5. Rath GK, Sharma DN, Shukla NK. Surgical resection with and without chemotherapy in oesophageal cancer. Lancet 2002;360(9340):1174 [author reply: 1175].
6. Allum WH, Stenning SP, Bancewicz J, et al. Long-term results of a randomized trial of surgery with or without preoperative chemotherapy in esophageal cancer. J Clin Oncol 2009;27(30):5062–7.
7. Cunningham D, Allum WH, Stenning SP, et al. Perioperative chemotherapy versus surgery alone for resectable gastroesophageal cancer. N Engl J Med 2006; 355(1):11–20.
8. Ychou M, Boige V, Pignon JP, et al. Perioperative chemotherapy compared with surgery alone for resectable gastroesophageal adenocarcinoma: an FNCLCC and FFCD multicenter phase III trial. J Clin Oncol 2011;29(13):1715–21.
9. Al-Batran SE, Hofheinz RD, Pauligk C, et al. Histopathological regression after neoadjuvant docetaxel, oxaliplatin, fluorouracil, and leucovorin versus epirubicin, cisplatin, and fluorouracil or capecitabine in patients with resectable gastric or gastro-oesophageal junction adenocarcinoma (FLOT4-AIO): results from the phase 2 part of a multicentre, open-label, randomised phase 2/3 trial. Lancet Oncol 2016;17(12):1697–708.
10. van Hagen P, Hulshof MC, van Lanschot JJ, et al. Preoperative chemoradiotherapy for esophageal or junctional cancer. N Engl J Med 2012;366(22):2074–84.
11. Shapiro J, van Lanschot JJB, Hulshof M, et al. Neoadjuvant chemoradiotherapy plus surgery versus surgery alone for oesophageal or junctional cancer (CROSS): long-term results of a randomised controlled trial. Lancet Oncol 2015;16(9):1090–8.
12. Walsh TN, Noonan N, Hollywood D, et al. A comparison of multimodal therapy and surgery for esophageal adenocarcinoma. N Engl J Med 1996;335(7):462–7.
13. Tepper J, Krasna MJ, Niedzwiecki D, et al. Phase III trial of trimodality therapy with cisplatin, fluorouracil, radiotherapy, and surgery compared with surgery alone for esophageal cancer: CALGB 9781. J Clin Oncol 2008;26(7):1086–92.
14. Klevebro F, Alexandersson von Dobeln G, Wang N, et al. A randomized clinical trial of neoadjuvant chemotherapy versus neoadjuvant chemoradiotherapy for

cancer of the oesophagus or gastro-oesophageal junction. Ann Oncol 2016; 27(4):660–7.

15. Burmeister BH, Thomas JM, Burmeister EA, et al. Is concurrent radiation therapy required in patients receiving preoperative chemotherapy for adenocarcinoma of the oesophagus? A randomised phase II trial. Eur J Cancer 2011;47(3):354–60.

16. Stahl M, Walz MK, Stuschke M, et al. Phase III comparison of preoperative chemotherapy compared with chemoradiotherapy in patients with locally advanced adenocarcinoma of the esophagogastric junction. J Clin Oncol 2009; 27(6):851–6.

17. Spicer JD, Stiles BM, Sudarshan M, et al. Preoperative chemoradiation therapy versus chemotherapy in patients undergoing modified en bloc esophagectomy for locally advanced esophageal adenocarcinoma: is radiotherapy beneficial? Ann Thorac Surg 2016;101(4):1262–9 [discussion: 1969–70].

18. Sjoquist KM, Burmeister BH, Smithers BM, et al. Survival after neoadjuvant chemotherapy or chemoradiotherapy for resectable oesophageal carcinoma: an updated meta-analysis. Lancet Oncol 2011;12(7):681–92.

19. Reynolds JV, Preston SR, O'Neill B, et al. ICORG 10-14: NEOadjuvant trial in Adenocarcinoma of the oEsophagus and oesophagoGastric junction International Study (Neo-AEGIS). BMC Cancer 2017;17(1):401.

20. Leong T, Smithers BM, Michael M, et al. TOPGEAR: a randomised phase III trial of perioperative ECF chemotherapy versus preoperative chemoradiation plus perioperative ECF chemotherapy for resectable gastric cancer (an international, intergroup trial of the AGITG/TROG/EORTC/NCIC CTG). BMC Cancer 2015;15: 532.

21. Hoeppner J, Lordick F, Brunner T, et al. ESOPEC: prospective randomized controlled multicenter phase III trial comparing perioperative chemotherapy (FLOT protocol) to neoadjuvant chemoradiation (CROSS protocol) in patients with adenocarcinoma of the esophagus (NCT02509286). BMC Cancer 2016;16: 503.

22. Stahl M, Stuschke M, Lehmann N, et al. Chemoradiation with and without surgery in patients with locally advanced squamous cell carcinoma of the esophagus. J Clin Oncol 2005;23(10):2310–7.

23. Bedenne L, Michel P, Bouche O, et al. Chemoradiation followed by surgery compared with chemoradiation alone in squamous cancer of the esophagus: FFCD 9102. J Clin Oncol 2007;25(10):1160–8.

24. Markar S, Gronnier C, Duhamel A, et al. Salvage surgery after chemoradiotherapy in the management of esophageal cancer: is it a viable therapeutic option? J Clin Oncol 2015;33(33):3866–73.

25. Noordman BJ, Wijnhoven BPL, Lagarde SM, et al. Neoadjuvant chemoradiotherapy plus surgery versus active surveillance for oesophageal cancer: a stepped-wedge cluster randomised trial. BMC Cancer 2018;18(1):142.

26. Lordick F, Ott K, Krause BJ, et al. PET to assess early metabolic response and to guide treatment of adenocarcinoma of the oesophagogastric junction: the MUNICON phase II trial. Lancet Oncol 2007;8(9):797–805.

27. Ott K, Fink U, Becker K, et al. Prediction of response to preoperative chemotherapy in gastric carcinoma by metabolic imaging: results of a prospective trial. J Clin Oncol 2003;21(24):4604–10.

28. Ott K, Weber WA, Lordick F, et al. Metabolic imaging predicts response, survival, and recurrence in adenocarcinomas of the esophagogastric junction. J Clin Oncol 2006;24(29):4692–8.

29. Mariette C, Dahan L, Mornex F, et al. Surgery alone versus chemoradiotherapy followed by surgery for stage I and II esophageal cancer: final analysis of randomized controlled phase III trial FFCD 9901. J Clin Oncol 2014;32(23):2416–22.

30. Markar SR, Gronnier C, Pasquer A, et al. Role of neoadjuvant treatment in clinical T2N0M0 oesophageal cancer: results from a retrospective multi-center European study. Eur J Cancer 2016;56:59–68.

31. Speicher PJ, Ganapathi AM, Englum BR, et al. Induction therapy does not improve survival for clinical stage T2N0 esophageal cancer. J Thorac Oncol 2014;9(8):1195–201.

32. Martin JT, Worni M, Zwischenberger JB, et al. The role of radiation therapy in resected T2 N0 esophageal cancer: a population-based analysis. Ann Thorac Surg 2013;95(2):453–8.

33. Ilson DH, van Hillegersberg R. Management of patients with adenocarcinoma or squamous cancer of the esophagus. Gastroenterology 2018;154(2):437–51.

34. Crabtree TD, Yacoub WN, Puri V, et al. Endoscopic ultrasound for early stage esophageal adenocarcinoma: implications for staging and survival. Ann Thorac Surg 2011;91(5):1509–15 [discussion: 1515–6].

35. Stiles BM, Mirza F, Coppolino A, et al. Clinical T2-T3N0M0 esophageal cancer: the risk of node positive disease. Ann Thorac Surg 2011;92(2):491–6 [discussion: 496–8].

Management of Early Stage Gastric and Gastroesophageal Junction Malignancies

Feredun S. Azari, MD, Robert E. Roses, MD*

KEYWORDS

- Early stage gastric cancer (ESGC) • Gastrectomy • EMR • ESD • H. pylori
- Gastroesophageal junction (GEJ) cancer • Barret's esophagus

KEY POINTS

- Gastric cancer is one of most common malignancies worldwide.
- Screening improves the detection of early stage gastric cancer, which has a greater than 90% 5-year survival rate.
- Early stage gastric cancer that meets the standard or expanded criteria can be treated using endoscopic mucosal resection and endoscopic submucosal dissection.
- Laparoscopic- or robotic- assisted gastrectomy and pylorus-preserving gastrectomy are viable treatment options with comparable outcomes to gold-standard surgical management in appropriately selected patients.
- Diagnosis and management of gastroesophageal cancers are based on staging and classification by either Siewert or recent American Joint Committee on Cancer guidelines.

CASE PRESENTATION

A 70-year-old woman with Lynch syndrome as well as significant medical comorbidities including coronary artery disease and diabetes mellitus was presented to the gastroenterologist for evaluation of a fundic gastric polyp found on surveillance endoscopy. She underwent endoscopic mucosal resection of the lesion with biopsy results revealing adenocarcinoma invading into the lamina propria with lymphovascular invasion extending to the lateral margins but with negative deep margins. She subsequently underwent repeat endoscopy, which showed postintervention scar. Multiple biopsies from the site were taken with inconclusive results. Given the suspicion for residual microscopic disease, she was referred for surgical consultation (**Fig. 1**).

The authors have nothing to disclose.
Department of Surgery, Hospital of the University of Pennsylvania, 3400 Spruce Street, 4 Silverstein Pavilion, Philadelphia, PA 19104, USA
* Corresponding author.
E-mail address: Robert.roses@uphs.upenn.edu

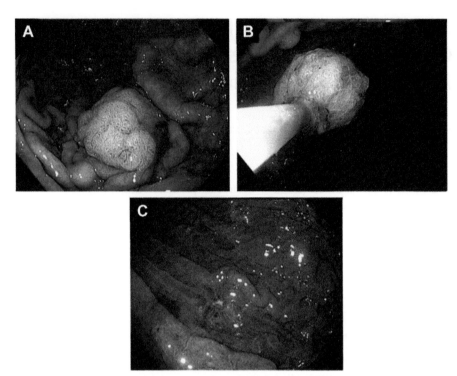

Fig. 1. (*A*) Polyp identified on the gastric fundus. (*B*) EMR of the gastric polyp. (*C*) Follow-up endoscopy after pathology revealed T1a disease with positive lateral margins demonstrating a scar.

INTRODUCTION

In the United States, gastric cancer accounts for approximately 26,000 new cases, and 10,000 deaths annually[1]; it comprises only 1.5% of all new cancer diagnoses and 1.8% of all cancer-related deaths. Worldwide, however, gastric cancer is a dominant case of cancer-related morbidity and mortality; it is the fourth most common cancer and the second leading cause of cancer death.[2] The burden of disease is highest in Asian, Latin American, and Eastern European countries.[2,3] Rates of new stomach cancer cases have been decreasing 1.5% on average each year over the last 10 years. Death rates have been decreasing 2.3% on average each year during the period from 2006 to 2015.[4,5] This phenomenon is explained, in part, by the identification of *Helicobacter pylori* infection as a major risk factor, which is thought to affect up to 50% of people worldwide, and the availability of effective antimicrobial therapy.[6] Infection by the bacteria may lead to chronic inflammation and atrophic gastritis. Atrophic gastritis can lead to intestinal metaplasia, a precursor for dysplastic changes and gastric cancer.[7] Environmental exposures such as pickled foods, salts, nitrosamines, and smoking have also been implicated in the development of gastric cancer; this may further explain the disproportionate incidence of disease in Asian countries compared with the West.[8] Another precursor to gastric malignancy, particularly in the west, is autoimmune metaplastic atrophic gastritis (AMAG).[9,10] In this chronic inflammatory condition, immune-mediated destruction of parietal cells leads to progressive loss of acid secretion and intrinsic factor. Patients with long-standing disease present with signs and symptoms of pernicious anemia. As the name implies AMAG, may manifest itself with metaplastic changes in the fundus and the body and affected patients have a 3-fold or greater increased relative risk of developing gastric adenocarcinoma.[9,10]

Risk factors for the development of gastric cancer in the cardia and noncardia regions of the stomach are different. Indeed, multiple studies have suggested that the risk of adenocarcinoma of the lower esophagus and gastroesophageal junction (GEJ) is reduced in individuals with confirmed *H pylori* infection. In contrast, gastric cancer of the cardia has been linked to gastroesophageal reflux disease and obesity.[11] This dichotomy has been ascribed to *H pylori*-induced gastric atrophy, which in turn decreases production of acid, decreasing inflammation in the cardia, GEJ, and lower esophagus.[5] Squamous cell carcinoma of the esophagus accounts for 90% of the newly diagnosed cases worldwide. However, diagnosis of esophageal adenocarcinoma is increasing, particularly in Western countries, and typically involves the distal esophagus or the GEJ.[12-15] The main risk factors for developing esophageal and GEJ cancers are gastroesophageal reflux disease (GERD), smoking, and obesity. Chronic GERD leads to the development of Barrett's esophagus (BE), metaplastic transformation of normal squamous epithelium to columnar epithelium.[12] These metaplastic changes lead to a sequence of dysplasia and neoplasia. There have been multiple population studies looking at progression of BE to high-grade dysplasia and adenocarcinoma, demonstrating an annual risk of progression to carcinoma of 0.9% to 1.0%.[12,13]

DEFINITION OF EARLY STAGE DISEASE
Early Stage Gastric Cancer

The most frequently invoked definition of early stage gastric cancer (ESGC) was initially proposed in early 1970s by Tadashige Murakami.[14] ESGC is defined as cancer in which the depth of invasion is limited to the submucosal layer of the stomach on histologic examination, regardless of lymph node status.[14] Despite the widespread acceptance of this definition, the exclusion of lymph node status has been contested.[15] In contrast to the high disease burden and poor prognosis associated with advanced stage of disease, ESGC has a favorable prognosis. In the United States, stage IA (mucosa or submucosa with no nodal involvement) disease is associated with a 94% 5-year survival (**Table 1**).[16,17] Thus, early diagnosis and treatment are of paramount importance. The low overall incidence of gastric cancer in Western countries explains the limited enthusiasm for aggressive screening programs. In contrast, in regions of the world with highest gastric cancer incidence, screening programs have been implemented and have effectively led to earlier diagnosis.[18] For example, in Japan, average-risk adults older than 40 years should undergo annual screening

Table 1 American Cancer Society gastric cancer 5-year observed survival rates	
Stage	**5-Year Observed Survival**
Stage IA	94%
Stage IB	88%
Stage IIA	82%
Stage IIB	68%
Stage IIIA	54%
Stage IIIB	36%
Stage IIIC	18%

with double-contrast barium and endoscopy. In Korea, upper endoscopy is recommended biannually in the same age group.[19] Approximately 50% of cases in Japan meet criteria for ESGC, compared with 15% in Europe.[20] In Korea, more than 60% of cases meet criteria for ESGC. Outcomes reported in 2009 and 2013 indicated 69% and 43% 5-year survival rates, respectively. This improvement in outcome was attributable to implementation of screening.[21,22]

Gastroesophageal Junction Cancer

Early esophageal cancers are defined as Tis (high-grade dysplasia) or T1 tumors. T1 tumors are further characterized as T1a (mucosa) and T1b (submucosa) depending on the depth of invasion.[23] GEJ cancers pose a dilemma given discreet paradigms for the staging and management of esophageal and gastric cancers. The higher frequency of BE in the United States confers an increased risk for distal esophageal and GEJ adenocarcinoma, which in the East are often classified as gastric cancer.[24] These tumors often share the same risk factors as esophageal adenocarcinoma, such as obesity, GERD, and tobacco use. Tumors of the cardia may share features of both types of carcinomas.[25] In 2012, the International Union Against Cancer recommended that GEJ tumors, irrespective of location, should be staged as esophageal cancers.[26] Notwithstanding this, treatment can include esophagogastrectomy (via transhiatal, thoracoabdominal, or combined abdominal and thoracic approaches) or extended transabdominal total gastrectomy with D2 lymphadenectomy, with most series failing to show a survival benefit for one operative approach over another.[27] Given the varied opinions on this matter, the anatomic classification proposed in the 1980s by Siewert and colleagues[28] has gained popularity and affords a convenient vocabulary with which to describe these lesions. In this classification system, type I lesions are adenocarcinomas of the distal esophagus, which usually arises from an area of intestinal metaplasia of the esophagus (ie, BE) and may infiltrate the esophagogastric junction from above; the tumor epicenter is located 1 cm above the GEJ. Type II lesions are true carcinomas of the cardia arising at the esophagogastric junction; the tumor epicenter is located 1 to 2 cm below the GEJ. Type III lesions are subcardial gastric carcinomas that infiltrates the esophagogastric junction and distal esophagus from below; the tumor epicenter is located more than 2 cm below the GEJ.[29,30] The American Joint Committee on Cancer (AJCC) has provided a clear distinction between esophageal and gastric cancers in order to classify tumors whose epicenter is in the distal esophagus or within the proximal 2 cm of stomach of which the mass protrudes into the GEJ or esophagus as an esophageal carcinoma. If the epicenter of the mass is more than 2 cm distal to and does not extend into the GEJ then it is classified as the gastric carcinoma.[16,31]

SURGICAL TREATMENT OPTIONS FOR EARLY STAGE GASTRIC CANCER
Traditional Surgical Approach

Operative resection with wide negative margins and regional nodal assessment remains the standard approach to the management of gastric cancer, including early stage disease. Subtotal or total gastrectomy is associated with 98% 5-year recurrence free survival in ESGC.[32] Extent and type of surgical resection depends on anatomic location. National Comprehensive Cancer Network recommends a 4-cm tumor-free margin and assessment of at least 16 lymph nodes.[4,33] In practice, tumors that reside in the upper third of the stomach, which include the Siewert type II and III GEJ cancers, and diffuse-type gastric cancers are managed with total gastrectomy with esophagojejunal reconstruction.[34] More distal tumors can be managed with subtotal distal gastrectomy (SDG) and gastrojejunal or gastroduodenal anastomosis. In either circumstance, regional nodes (left and right gastric, left and right gastroomental arteries, celiac artery, proximal splenic artery, and common hepatic artery) are removed.[35] Distal splenic artery lymph nodes and splenic hilar lymph nodes are also removed in conjunction with total gastrectomy.

Reconstruction options for SDG include Billroth I, Billroth II, and Roux-en-Y techniques. Regardless of the reconstruction option chosen, the goals of surgery are maintenance of function, minimization of postoperative morbidity, and satisfactory oncologic resection. Billroth I preserves physiologic alimentary tract continuity but may limit clearance of distal tumors or associates with anastomotic tension if the gastric remnant is smaller. Billroth II gastrojejunostomy compared with Billroth I is technically easier and can be done with minimal tension on the anastomosis. However, this type of reconstruction predisposes to complications such as bile reflux gastritis and afferent loop syndrome. Roux-en-Y gastrojejunostomy on the other hand minimizes gastroduodenal reflux but is more time consuming. Meta-analyses of Billroth I versus Billroth II versus Roux-en-Y suggest that Roux-en-Y reconstruction offers better clinical outcomes with less frequent reflux symptoms and esophagitis.[36,37]

Reconstruction after total gastrectomy usually entails Roux-en-Y esophagojejunostomy.[38] Some data support the use of jejunal reservoir as it may offer better functional and quality of life outcomes, at least in the early months to years following surgery.[39] In a randomized controlled trial (RCT) of 138 patients observed over a 12-year period, Fein and colleagues[40] found that patients undergoing Roux-en-Y reconstruction with a pouch had an improved quality of life and return to preoperative baseline within 2 years of index operation compared with those who did not have a pouch reconstruction. This was further corroborated by a recent meta-analysis of 17 randomized and 8 observational studies conducted by Syn and associates, which showed pouch formation improving long-term functional as well as nutritional outcomes without greater perioperative morbidity.[41]

Regardless of the choice of operation, complications associated with traditional surgical approach are not trivial. In one study of 2580 patients from a large national database, patients who underwent gastrectomy had a morbidity rate of 23.6% and 4.1% 30-day mortality rate. Serious morbidity and mortality were significantly higher in the total gastrectomy group than the partial gastrectomy group.[42] In a study by Bartlett and associates of a large US cohort undergoing total gastrectomy, 36% of patients experienced a complication and 4.7% of patients died within 30 days of operation.[43] Moreover, these studies do not address the long-term impact of gastrectomy on quality of life. All reconstructive approaches lead to alterations in eating habits and nutritional absorption. Such outcomes have motivated efforts to spare morbidity, particularly in patients with early stage disease.

MINIMALLY INVASIVE SURGICAL MANAGEMENT OF EARLY STAGE GASTRIC CANCER

Improvements in laparoscopic technology and increased surgeon expertise have led to wider acceptance of laparoscopy in the management of gastric cancer, particularly in Asia. Since its description in 1994, multiple RCTs have been performed in Korea and Japan comparing laparoscopic versus open gastrectomy for ESGC.[44,45] One of the first, reported by Kitano and associates in 2002, found that laparoscopic distal gastrectomy was associated with significantly decreased intraoperative blood loss, length of hospital stay, and pain compared with the open approach.[46] Recently published prospective studies and meta-analyses affirm the feasibility of minimally invasive gastrectomy.[47–50] In 2016, the Korean Laparoscopic Gastrointestinal Group published the results of a phase III prospective multicenter RCT demonstrating that a[45,47,48,50] laparoscopic approach was associated with decreased length of hospital stay, blood loss, and complication rate. Survival rates between the open and laparoscopic group were similar.[49] One meta-analysis that included 5 RCTs and 17 non-RCTs compared more than 3000 patients who underwent laparoscopic distal gastrectomy versus an open approach. The laparoscopic approach was associated with similar lymph node assessment, decreased intraoperative blood loss, decreased postoperative analgesia requirements, and reduced hospital stay.[51] The investigators concluded that under experienced surgical hands, laparoscopic approach is practical and may afford faster post-op recovery in ESGC.

Data from the West on minimally invasive gastrectomy consist largely of retrospective single institutional studies. A prospective RCT that compared 59 patients of whom 30 underwent laparoscopic intervention found that laparoscopic group had similar short- and long-term oncologic outcome compared with the open group; however, the laparoscopic group had reduced blood loss, decreased hospital stay, and earlier initiation of oral intake.[48] A large case-matched retrospective study from Memorial Sloan Kettering and City of Hope showed similar oncologic outcomes after minimally invasive and open surgery but decreased length of stay and early and late postoperative complications after minimally invasive gastrectomy.[52,53] It remains uncertain whether outcomes achieved with minimally invasive gastrectomy at selected high-volume centers are more broadly reproducible in the United States. A retrospective analysis drawing on the National Cancer Database showed that minimally invasive gastrectomy was associated with shorter hospital stay, equivalent lymph node examination, and superior rates of R0 resection compared with an open approach.[54] However, outcome disparities were noted at academic compared with nonacademic and higher volume compared with lower volume centers.

ENDOSCOPIC TREATMENT OF EARLY STAGE GASTRIC CANCER

Patients in whom staging reveals only mucosal (T1a) disease are candidates for endoscopic mucosal resection (EMR) and endoscopic submucosal dissection (ESD) supported by multiple studies demonstrating low rates of lymph node metastasis in disease confined to the mucosal or lamina propria.[55] However, it should be noted that, to date, there are no RCTs comparing endoscopic treatment of ESGC versus the standard surgical approach with regional lymphadenectomy.[56] EMR and ESD are optimal for intestinal (localized) gastric cancer types and should not replace standard surgical management for diffuse type gastric cancer. There are established standard criteria for endoscopic intervention founded on a low risk of recurrence (**Box 1**), which include lesions that are intramucosal, well-differentiated,

---

Box 1
Standard criteria for endoscopic resection of gastric cancer

Intramucosal lesion

Well-differentiated intestinal type (vs diffuse type)

Less than 2 cm in size

No evidence of neoplastic ulcer

No evidence of lymphovascular involvement

Negative margins (deep and horizontal)

of the intestinal type, less than 2 cm in size, nonulcerated, and without evidence of lymphovascular invasion.[57]

A variety of techniques have been developed since the original EMR technique was described in Japan by Murakami and colleagues. However, typical elements of EMR include submucosal injection of hypertonic fluid that allows lifting of the lesion and then removal using a snare. In a study from Uedo and associates, patients who underwent EMR had 5- and 10-year overall survival rates of 84% and 64%, respectively. Disease-specific survival at 10-year follow-up was 99%.[58] Similar findings were observed in other East Asian centers who have adopted EMR as a treatment of choice in ESGC.[57,59] Despite the feasibility of technique, EMR has a tendency to fragment tumors larger than 2.0 cm, resulting in incomplete histologic evaluation and increased risk of local recurrence reported as high as 2% to 35% when compared with en-bloc resection.[57] A recent 10-year follow-up study from Japan showed that tumor size larger than 2 cm is an independent risk factor for local recurrence.[60] Similar findings were reported from a European trial where the local recurrence rate was 29%; all recurrences were treated with repeat endoscopy.[61] Patients with submucosal invasion, lymphovascular invasion, and positive vertical margins are generally referred for surgery. In a study published by Nagano and associates, the investigators suggested that patients with only positive lateral margins should undergo endoscopic surveillance, whereas those found to have submucosal invasions and positive vertical margins should be referred for gastrectomy.[62]

ESD has emerged as a technique to allow en-bloc resection of mucosal and submucosal lesions irrespective of size. Basic steps of ESD include circumferential marking of the lesion, submucosal dye injection, lateral dissection using specialized knives, and *en bloc* retrieval. Because the procedure is technically challenging, ESD is generally performed at specialized centers. Studies comparing ESD versus EMR have shown that ESD is more likely to allow complete histologic excision and is associated with a lower recurrence rate but a higher risk of perforation.[63] In a retrospective analysis comparing ESD with EMR, ESD achieved greater *en bloc* resection rates but did not improve survival for tumors larger than 2 cm.[64] ESD had fewer complications while maintaining similar survival compared with traditional surgical resection. These findings support investigating endoscopic approaches for ESGC as a viable alternative to surgery.[65]

More penetrative lesions with higher risk of occult nodal disease are not well treated with local excision and patient selection remains a critical determinant of outcome. Notwithstanding, there has been an increasing effort to expand inclusion criteria for endoscopic treatment of ESGC.[66] Proposed expanded criteria (**Box 2**) include differentiated mucosal tumors of any size without ulceration, mucosal tumors less than 3 cm with ulceration, undifferentiated mucosal tumors less than 2 cm without ulceration, and submucosal tumors less than 3 cm confined to the upper 0.5 mm of the submucosa without lymphovascular invasion.

Box 2
Expanded criteria for endoscopic resection of gastric cancer

Differentiated mucosal tumors without ulceration (any size)

Differentiated mucosal tumors with ulceration (<3 cm)

Undifferentiated mucosal tumors less than 2 cm without ulceration

Submucosal lesions less than 3 cm confined to the upper 0.5 mm of the submucosa without lymphovascular invasion

Early reports suggested that ESD was a reasonable alternative approach for lesions meeting the expanded criteria. However, a recent meta-analysis indicated that patients who meet the expanded criteria are at higher risk for lymph node metastasis versus the standard criteria.[67] Expanded criteria have been adopted at selected centers but are considered investigational at the current time.

FUNCTION-PRESERVING AND MINIMALLY INVASIVE SURGICAL OPTIONS FOR EARLY STAGE GASTRIC CANCER
Pylorus Preserving Gastrectomy (Central Gastrectomy)

Given the short- and longer-term morbidity associated with traditional surgical approaches for gastric cancer, surgical techniques that mitigate those risks have been explored. These function-preserving techniques attempt to minimize bile reflux, dumping syndrome, and other functional symptoms that affect quality of life. One such option is pylorus-preserving gastrectomy (PPG). PPG has been used for tumors in the middle third of the stomach without evidence of lymph node metastasis. The central portion of the stomach is resected and a gastrogastrostomy is created. More limited regional lymphadenectomy is performed, preserving the nodes around the pylorus (level 5 and 6) in order to spare hepatic branches of the vagus nerve (level 5) and the infrapyloric vessels (level 6).[68,69] PPG should be performed only when the risk of lymph node involvement is low after adequate staging and diagnosis. The Japanese gastric cancer guidelines recommend PPG for clinical T1N0M0 tumors that are at least 4 cm away from the pylorus.[70] The benefits of PPG, when compared with DG, include the lower incidence of dumping syndrome, bile reflux, and gallstone formation as well as less impact on nutritional parameters.[68,71,72] The most common functional complication associated with PPG is gastric stasis, which may be managed with dilation and stents. Five-year survival amongst appropriately selected patients with PPG is comparable to that achieved with traditional subtotal gastrectomy.[68]

Local Resection and Sentinel Lymph Biopsy

Standard gastric resections even with modified approaches are associated with variety of postgastrectomy syndromes and a decrement in quality of life.[73] In light of this, many groups have approached localized superficial lesions with more limited or local gastric resection. Generally, full-thickness local excision is most appropriate for lesions that would meet criteria for endoscopic intervention.[74] Local resection options include purely laparoscopic, endoscopic full-thickness, and combined laparoscopic endoscopic approaches.

Local operative techniques may allow R0 resection while sparing the morbidity associated with more extensive resection. Even in the setting of difficult laparoscopic resection, particularly for endophytic lesions, cooperative laparoendoscopic approaches are sometimes feasible.[75] The endoscope may be used to localize and dissect circumferentially around the tumor or mass in a submucosal layer. Laparoscopy is used to dissect the seromuscular layer. The tumor is subsequently removed laparoscopically, and the gastric defect is closed using a stapling device or with intracorporeal suturing. Encouraging results from such approaches have been reported in various small studies demonstrating minimal intraoperative blood loss and postoperative morbidity and mortality.[76–78]

In the setting of ESGC, subtotal or total gastrectomy is rationalized, in part, by the risk of occult regional nodal disease. Given the low risk of regional nodal disease in patients with T1 tumors in particular, many patients are overtreated by such approaches. Even tumors confined to submucosa (T1b) carries a less than 20% chance of lymph node metastasis. Better techniques to preoperatively identify the presence or absence of lymph node metastasis accurately could increase the proportion of early gastric cancer approachable with local excision. Drawing on an experience with tracer-guided selective lymphadenectomy in breast cancer and melanoma skin cancer (ie, sentinel lymphadenectomy), several investigators have explored sentinel lymph node navigation (SLN) for gastric cancer. SLN uses a tracer such as isosulfan blue, patent blue, or indocyanine green. The tracer is injected around the tumor endoscopically and dye-stained lymphatics can then be visualized. Selective removal of early draining lymph nodes with pathologic assessment may distinguish patients with low risk of nodal involvement (negative sentinel node) from those who require more extensive regional nodal dissection (positive sentinel node).[79] A theoretic limitation of this approach for stomach tumors is the rich and redundant lymphatic drainage, which may increase the risk of inaccurate staging. Notwithstanding, recent prospective studies of SLN suggested good sensitivity and accuracy in smaller tumors. However, it is associated with a false-negative rate as high as 46%. Thus, the concept of SLN for ESGC remains investigational.[80]

Ablative Treatment

For patients who have lesions that are amenable to curative intent resections but are unable to undergo surgical or endoscopic interventions (usually owing to prohibitive medical comorbidities), Kitamura and associates described the use of argon plasma coagulation.[81] The patients included in the study had advanced liver disease, renal disease, and coagulopathy. Average time to progression from ESGC to advanced stage disease was 37 months.[82]

Special Populations

Certain genetic risk factors such as CDH1 mutation, which predisposes for hereditary diffuse gastric cancer (HDGC), fall outside of conventional management of ESGC, even in early disease. Affected patients have a 67% to 83% chance of developing diffuse type gastric cancer by age 80 years, with women having higher predilection.[4] Apart from gastric cancer, women afflicted with the genetic mutation carry an increased risk of developing lobular type breast cancer.[83] Management of patients with HDGC depends on the knowledge of individual's CDH1 mutation status. Guidelines recommend that those with pathogenic CDH1 mutation who are older than 20 years should undergo prophylactic total gastrectomy regardless of endoscopic findings. Those without genetic testing but with strong family history undergo endoscopic screening, whereas those with known mutation who choose not to pursue surgery or are younger than 20 years of age should undergo surveillance.[4,34,83] The optimal frequency of endoscopic surveillance is not known, but given the current expertise, it should be at least performed annually at centers with experience in treating and counseling these patients. Gastric cancer has also been found in other hereditary cancer syndromes, which include gastric adenocarcinoma and proximal polyposis of the stomach syndrome, Li-Fraumeni syndrome, familial adenomatous polyposis, Lynch syndrome, and Peutz-Jeghers syndrome.[4]

SURGICAL TREATMENT OPTIONS FOR GASTROESOPHAGEAL JUNCTION DISEASE

Despite the lack of a clear anatomic demarcation between the GEJ and the stomach, malignancies in these regions are often treated differently. Both the AJCC and Siewert have proposed distance cutoffs to help differentiate amongst the two. Broadly speaking, Siewert I and II tumors are often managed as esophageal carcinoma. The eighth edition of the AJCC guidelines proposed that tumors with epicenters 2 cm from the GEJ be managed as stomach cancers.[16]

Until recently, definitive surgical management with lymphadenectomy was the gold standard for management of esophageal malignancy, even with early stage disease. More recent evidence indicates that the operations commonly used in this setting are associated with increased short-term morbidity and mortality without an obvious long-term benefit.[84] Given this, surgical approach has been advocated T1b and greater disease. Surgical treatment for esophageal neoplasia includes transhiatal, transthoracic, and three-hole (McKeown) esophagectomies. The procedures differ with respect to the location and number of incisions as well as the site of anastomosis to the gastric conduit. Transhiatal approach usually uses a laparotomy or laparoscopy and a left neck incision where the anastomosis is created. The transthoracic approach, also known as Ivor Lewis esophagectomy, typically uses laparotomy or laparoscopy and right thoracotomy or thoracoscopy. Prospective studies have failed to consistently demonstrate a significant difference between these operations with regard to oncologic outcomes.[85–90] Comparative studies have observed that long-term survival after transhiatal esophagectomy is equivalent to or better than that seen after transthoracic esophagectomy and the transhiatal approach is associated with a lower risk of perioperative mortality compared with the transthoracic approach.[88,91] Omloo and associates, on the other hand, in their 5-year RCT found that the transthoracic approach allowed for increased lymph node dissection and improved locoregional disease-free survival.[92]

In recent years, minimally invasive approaches to esophagectomy have been adopted to mitigate perioperative risk. Analysis of 18,673 esophagectomies over a 12-year period from England found that minimally invasive esophagectomy group had a similar mortality and length-of-stay outcomes when compared with an open approach.[93] Similar analysis of 4266 patients from the National Cancer Database in 2016 found that the laparoscopic approach was associated with increase in lymph node retrieval, shorter hospital stay, and similar 3-year survival outcomes compared with the open approach.[94] A retrospective comparative analysis of 130 patients by Tapias and associates from Massachusetts General Hospital reported that patients who underwent laparoscopic compared with open resection had decreased postoperative pulmonary complications with similar oncologic, 3- and 5-year survival rates.[95] With respect to technique, a study comparing 1000 patients who underwent minimally invasive esophagectomy with either McKeown or Ivor Lewis technique found that mortality, lymph node dissection, and postoperative outcomes were the same amongst the groups with statistically significant increase in recurrent laryngeal nerve injury with procedures involving a neck anastomosis.[90]

ENDOSCOPIC TREATMENT OPTIONS FOR EARLY STAGE GASTROESOPHAGEAL JUNCTION AND BARRETT'S ESOPHAGUS

As with tumors of the stomach, the risk of lymph node metastasis from GE junction and distal esophageal cancers correlates with depth of invasion of the tumor. In BE

Table 2
Treatment modalities for early stage gastroesophageal junction disease

Stage	Treatment Approach
Stage 0 and I (Tis and Tia) Barret's with High-grade dysplasia	EMR (first choice) Esophagectomy with lymphadenectomy (second choice) Definitive chemoradiotherapy if unable to undergo surgery or patient choice
T1b	Esophagectomy with lymphadenectomy

Data from Rustgi AK, El-Serag HB. Esophageal carcinoma. N Engl J Med 2014;371(26):2499–509.

with high-grade dysplasia, the risk of misdiagnosis with an early stage cancer with occult lymph node metastases is less than 1% and between 1% and 2% for T1a disease.[96] This risk increases to approximately 20% in disease that is found to penetrate the submucosa.[5] In lower-risk patients, local resection of disease can represent definitive therapy.[97] Options for local resection include EMR, ESD, radiofrequency ablation, cryotherapy, and free-hand mucosal resection. To date, there have not been RCTs comparing different endoscopic options with gold-standard surgical therapy, but there is consensus that all visible lesions have to be removed via EMR to assess depth of invasion, because staging techniques such as endoscopic ultrasound are poor at detecting difference between T1a and T1b disease (**Table 2**).[97]

A series looking at EMR as an approach for BE with HGD and T1a lesions reported by Pech and associates found that at 63 months there was 96.6% complete response with 21.5% recurrence rate but no death related to disease.[98] Prasad and associates performed a retrospective analysis of 178 patients comparing endoscopic and surgical treatment of T1a disease. Out of 132 patients who underwent endoscopic treatment had similar oncologic and survival outcomes when compared with surgical approach, but the endoscopic group was noted to have increased risk of metachronous lesions during a follow-up period.[99] Chennat and associates found similar results when using EMR in patients diagnosed with BE with high-grade dysplasia. In their study there was 96% remission rate, with 37% of patients developing symptomatic esophageal stenosis requiring multiple dilations.[100] Despite the current recommendations, analysis of 782 patients with early stage adenocarcinoma who underwent surgical resection has found that for T1a disease with poor differentiation or size larger than 2 cm, esophagectomy should be considered.[101] Thus, accurate staging and pathologic analysis is paramount.

Results of endoscopic intervention for T1b disease are less encouraging but in spite of the known risk of occult lymph node metastases, endoscopic management of T1b disease has increased by 4 times since 2004.[102] As expected, analysis by Ballard and associates found approximately 38% recurrence rate in those undergoing endoscopic therapy for T1b disease.[103] Despite these results, EMR and ESD could be suitable for certain subset of population. In a separate analysis from the NCDB, Newton and associates found that in patients with T1b tumors smaller than 2 cm, without lymphovascular invasion, endoscopic resection was associated with favorable outcomes.[101]

ESD is also a suitable option for early disease that meets criteria for endoscopic resection via EMR. ESD allows en-bloc resection of squamous cell cancer (SCC) lesions that are larger than 2 cm and may also be used for T1b tumors without lymphovascular invasion disease where EMR falls short and is associated with an increased risk of piecemeal extraction.[104] In a meta-analysis of ESD, en-bloc resection was achieved in 99% of cases and R0 resection was achieved in 90% of lesions smaller than 2.5 cm. The most common complications were esophageal stenosis (5%) and perforation (1%).[105] Another study looking at patients who underwent curative ESD found a 5-year survival of 100% with no metastatic recurrences.[106] The data for ESD are primarily from Asian countries and focuses on SCC and may not be generalizable to patients in the West.[107]

OTHER LOCAL TREATMENT MODALITIES FOR EARLY STAGE ESOPHAGEAL CANCER AND BARRETT'S ESOPHAGUS

Other local ablative therapies are available for the treatment of early stage esophageal disease and BE. Sometimes used in conjunction with EMR/ESD, these approaches allow treatment of longer segment BE. Therapies supported by evidence, albeit limited in some cases, include photodynamic therapy (PDT), argon plasma coagulation (APC), and radiofrequency ablation (RFA).

PDT involves intravenous injection of sodium salt of porphyrin, which has a tropism for neoplastic tissue and is stimulated at precise wavelength of 630 nm, which is done endoscopically. Studies of PDT with EMR indicate an 83% to 94% remission rate in the first year.[108,109] Complication associated with combination of PDT and EMR is esophageal stenosis and skin photosensitivity.

APC involves the use of a highly ionized argon jet to thermo-destruct the lesion of interest. In a study with long-term follow-up, patients with nondysplastic BE who underwent APC were not protected against cancer development.[110] RFA involves the use of high-frequency emitting electrodes that are either attached to an endoscope or a balloon or directly applied to the tissue of interest. RFA may be performed after EMR in order to allow analysis of depth of invasion; lesions with submucosal involvement should undergo operative management. One study analyzing RFA with and without EMR found that the combined technique was associated with complete eradication of dysplastic tissue in 94% of cases and metaplastic tissue in 88% of cases. RFA alone was associated with complete eradication of dysplastic tissue in 82.7% of cases and metaplastic tissue in 77.6% of cases. Complication rates were similar in both groups.[111]

CASE CONTINUED

Given the concern for residual microscopic disease on the positive lateral margins, low risk of occult nodal involvement, and complex medical comorbidities, the patient decided to forego subtotal gastric resection and was elected for cooperative laparoscopic and endoscopic full-thickness excision. During the procedure the clipped area from prior EMR was identified with the aid of an endoscope and elevated for identification in the peritoneal cavity by a laparoscope. The area of interest was mobilized and widely excised. Pathologic assessment revealed residual gastric adenoma with high-grade dysplasia adjacent to prior biopsy site with no residual carcinoma. Patient has been undergoing annual endoscopic surveillance without evidence of recurrence.

SUMMARY

Optimal treatment for ESGC requires accurate diagnosis and staging. Traditional surgical approaches remain the gold standards but early stage disease (T1) can be managed with endoscopic approaches such as EMR and ESD or more conservative resection. Adoption of these approaches in the West has been slow compared with the East where early stage disease is more frequently diagnosed. Increased utilization of these approaches may preserve quality of life without compromising oncologic outcomes and should be considered in appropriately selected patients.

REFERENCES

1. Esophageal cancer - cancer stat facts [Internet]. Available at: https://seer.cancer.gov/statfacts/html/esoph.html. Accessed August 22, 2018.
2. Luo G, Zhang Y, Guo P, et al. Global patterns and trends in stomach cancer incidence: age, period and birth cohort analysis. Int J Cancer 2017;141(7):1333–44.
3. Stomach cancer - cancer stat facts [Internet]. Available at: https://seer.cancer.gov/statfacts/html/stomach.html. Accessed June 3, 2018.
4. Van Cutsem E, Sagaert X, Topal B, et al. Gastric cancer. Lancet 2016;388(10060):2654–64.

5. Rustgi AK, El-Serag HB. Esophageal carcinoma. N Engl J Med 2014;371(26): 2499–509.

6. Bornschein J, Selgrad M, Warnecke M, et al. pylori infection is a key risk factor for proximal gastric cancer. Dig Dis Sci 2010;55(11):3124–31.

7. Park YH, Kim N. Review of atrophic gastritis and intestinal metaplasia as a premalignant lesion of gastric cancer. J Cancer Prev 2015;20(1):25–40.

8. Wroblewski LE, Peek RM, Wilson KT. Helicobacter pylori and gastric cancer: factors that modulate disease risk. Clin Microbiol Rev 2010;23(4):713–39.

9. Autoimmune metaplastic atrophic gastritis - gastrointestinal disorders [Internet]. Merck Manuals Professional Edition. Available at: https://www.merckmanuals. com/professional/gastrointestinal-disorders/gastritis-and-peptic-ulcer-disease/ autoimmune-metaplastic-atrophic-gastritis. Accessed September 11, 2018.

10. Vannella L, Lahner E, Annibale B. Risk for gastric neoplasias in patients with chronic atrophic gastritis: a critical reappraisal. World J Gastroenterol 2012; 18(12):1279–85.

11. Karimi P, Islami F, Anandasabapathy S, et al. Gastric cancer: descriptive epidemiology, risk factors, screening, and prevention. Cancer Epidemiol Biomark Prev 2014;23(5):700–13.

12. Schoofs N, Bisschops R, Prenen H. Progression of Barrett's esophagus toward esophageal adenocarcinoma: an overview. Ann Gastroenterol 2017;30(1):1–6.

13. de Jonge PJF, van Blankenstein M, Looman CWN, et al. Risk of malignant progression in patients with Barrett's oesophagus: a Dutch nationwide cohort study. Gut 2010;59(8):1030–6.

14. Murakami T. Early cancer of the stomach. World J Surg 1979;3(6):685–91.

15. Saragoni L. Upgrading the definition of early gastric cancer: better staging means more appropriate treatment. Cancer Biol Med 2015;12(4):355–61.

16. In H, Solsky I, Palis B, et al. Validation of the 8th edition of the AJCC TNM staging system for gastric cancer using the National Cancer Database. Ann Surg Oncol 2017;24(12):3683–91.

17. Stomach cancer survival rates [Internet]. Available at: https://www.cancer.org/ cancer/stomach-cancer/detection-diagnosis-staging/survival-rates.html. Accessed August 4, 2018.

18. Yamamoto M, Rashid OM, Wong J. Surgical management of gastric cancer: the East vs. West perspective. J Gastrointest Oncol 2015;6(1):79–88.

19. Bickenbach K, Strong VE. Comparisons of gastric cancer treatments: East vs. West. J Gastric Cancer 2012;12(2):55–62.

20. Yoon H, Kim N. Diagnosis and management of high risk group for gastric cancer. Gut Liver 2015;9(1):5–17.

21. Choi IJ. Gastric cancer screening and diagnosis. Korean J Gastroenterol 2009; 54(2):67–76 [in Korean].

22. Cho E, Kang MH, Choi KS, et al. Cost-effectiveness outcomes of the national gastric cancer screening program in South Korea. Asian Pac J Cancer Prev 2013;14(4):2533–40.

23. Rice Thomas W, Gress Donna M, Patil Deepa T, et al. Cancer of the esophagus and esophagogastric junction—Major changes in the American Joint Committee on Cancer eighth edition cancer staging manual. CA Cancer J Clin 2017;67(4): 304–17.

24. Kim GH, Liang PS, Bang SJ, et al. Screening and surveillance for gastric cancer in the United States: is it needed? Gastrointest Endosc 2016;84(1):18–28.

25. von Rahden BHA, Feith M, Stein HJ. Carcinoma of the cardia: classification as esophageal or gastric cancer? Int J Colorectal Dis 2005;20(2):89–93.

26. Schuhmacher C, Novotny A, Feith M, et al. The new TNM classification of tumors of the esophagogastric junction. Surgical consequences. Chirurg 2012;83(1):23–30 [in German].

27. Barbour AP, Rizk NP, Gonen M, et al. Adenocarcinoma of the gastroesophageal junction. Ann Surg 2007;246(1):1–8.

28. Curtis NJ, Noble F, Bailey IS, et al. The relevance of the Siewert classification in the era of multimodal therapy for adenocarcinoma of the gastro-oesophageal junction. J Surg Oncol 2014;109(3):202–7.

29. Rüdiger Siewert J, Feith M, Werner M, et al. Adenocarcinoma of the esophago-gastric junction. Ann Surg 2000;232(3):353–61.

30. Siewert JR, Stein HJ, Feith M. Adenocarcinoma of the Esophago-Gastric junction. Scand J Surg 2006;95(4):260–9.

31. Edge SB, Compton CC. The American Joint Committee on cancer: the 7th edition of the AJCC cancer staging manual and the future of TNM. Ann Surg Oncol 2010;17(6):1471–4.

32. Youn HG, An JY, Choi MG, et al. Recurrence after curative resection of early gastric cancer. Ann Surg Oncol 2010;17(2):448–54.

33. NCCN stomach cancer guidelines [Internet]. Available at: https://www.nccn.org/patients/guidelines/stomach/files/assets/common/downloads/files/stomach.pdf. Accessed August 7, 2018.

34. Lynch HT, Silva E, Wirtzfeld D, et al. Hereditary diffuse gastric cancer: prophylactic surgical oncology implications. Surg Clin North Am 2008;88(4):759–78, vii.

35. Surgery for cancer of the stomach- ClinicalKey [Internet]. Available at: https://www.clinicalkey.com/#!/content/book/3-s2.0-B9780702049620000072?scrollTo=%23hl0000627. Accessed August 25, 2018.

36. Zong L, Chen P. Billroth I vs. Billroth II vs. Roux-en-Y following distal gastrectomy: a meta-analysis based on 15 studies. Hepatogastroenterology 2011;58(109):1413–24.

37. Buhl K, Schlag P, Herfarth C. Quality of life and functional results following different types of resection for gastric carcinoma. Eur J Surg Oncol 1990;16(4):404–9.

38. Total gastrectomy and gastrointestinal reconstruction - UpToDate [Internet]. Available at: https://www.uptodate.com/contents/total-gastrectomy-and-gastrointestinal-reconstruction. Accessed August 8, 2018.

39. El Halabi HM, Lawrence W. Clinical results of various reconstructions employed after total gastrectomy. J Surg Oncol 2007;97(2):186–92.

40. Fein M, Fuchs K-H, Thalheimer A, et al. Long-term benefits of Roux-en-Y pouch reconstruction after total gastrectomy: a randomized trial. Ann Surg 2008;247(5):759–65.

41. Syn NL, Wee I, Shabbir A, et al. Pouch versus no pouch following total gastrectomy: meta-analysis of randomized and non-randomized studies. Ann Surg 2019. Available at: https://journals.lww.com/annalsofsurgery/Abstract/publishahead/Pouch_Versus_No_Pouch_Following_Total_gastrectomy_.95344.aspx. Accessed February 8, 2019.

42. Papenfuss WA, Kukar M, Oxenberg J, et al. Morbidity and mortality associated with gastrectomy for gastric cancer. Ann Surg Oncol 2014;21(9):3008–14.

43. Bartlett EK, Roses RE, Kelz RR, et al. Morbidity and mortality after total gastrectomy for gastric malignancy using the American College of Surgeons National Surgical Quality Improvement Program database. Surgery 2014;156(2):298–304.

44. Russo A, Strong VE. Minimally invasive surgery for gastric cancer in USA: current status and future perspectives. Transl Gastroenterol Hepatol 2017;2:1–8. Available at: https://www.ncbi.nlm.nih.gov/pmc/articles/PMC5420518/.

45. Kim Y-W, Baik YH, Yun YH, et al. Improved quality of life outcomes after laparoscopy-assisted distal gastrectomy for early gastric cancer: results of a prospective randomized clinical trial. Ann Surg 2008;248(5):721–7.

46. Kitano S, Shiraishi N, Fujii K, et al. A randomized controlled trial comparing open vs laparoscopy-assisted distal gastrectomy for the treatment of early gastric cancer: an interim report. Surgery 2002;131(1 Suppl):S306–11.

47. Lee J-H, Han H-S, Lee J-H. A prospective randomized study comparing open vs laparoscopy-assisted distal gastrectomy in early gastric cancer: early results. Surg Endosc 2005;19(2):168–73.

48. Huscher CGS, Mingoli A, Sgarzini G, et al. Laparoscopic versus open subtotal gastrectomy for distal gastric cancer: five-year results of a randomized prospective trial. Ann Surg 2005;241(2):232–7.

49. Kim W, Kim H-H, Han S-U, et al. Decreased morbidity of laparoscopic distal gastrectomy compared with open distal gastrectomy for stage i gastric cancer: short-term outcomes from a multicenter randomized controlled trial (KLASS-01). Ann Surg 2016;263(1):28–35.

50. Kim H-H, Hyung WJ, Cho GS, et al. Morbidity and mortality of laparoscopic gastrectomy versus open gastrectomy for gastric cancer: an interim report–a phase III multicenter, prospective, randomized trial (KLASS Trial). Ann Surg 2010; 251(3):417–20.

51. Zeng Y-K, Yang Z-L, Peng J-S, et al. Laparoscopy-assisted versus open distal gastrectomy for early gastric cancer: evidence from randomized and non-randomized clinical trials. Ann Surg 2012;256(1):39–52.

52. Strong VE, Devaud N, Allen PJ, et al. Laparoscopic versus open subtotal gastrectomy for adenocarcinoma: a case-control study. Ann Surg Oncol 2009; 16(6):1507–13.

53. Guzman EA, Pigazzi A, Lee B, et al. Totally laparoscopic gastric resection with extended lymphadenectomy for gastric adenocarcinoma. Ann Surg Oncol 2009;16(8):2218–23.

54. Ecker BL, Datta J, McMillan MT, et al. Minimally invasive gastrectomy for gastric adenocarcinoma in the United States: utilization and short-term oncologic outcomes. J Surg Oncol 2015;112(6):616–21.

55. Songun I, Putter H, Kranenbarg EM, et al. Surgical treatment of gastric cancer: 15-year follow-up results of the randomised nationwide Dutch D1D2 trial. Lancet Oncol 2010;11(5):439–49.

56. Bennett C, Wang Y, Pan T. Endoscopic mucosal resection for early gastric cancer. Cochrane Database Syst Rev 2009;(4). CD004276. The Cochrane Library [Internet]. John Wiley & Sons, Ltd. Available at: http://cochranelibrary-wiley. com/doi/10.1002/14651858.CD004276.pub3/abstract. Accessed June 22, 2018.

57. Min YW, Min B-H, Lee JH, et al. Endoscopic treatment for early gastric cancer. World J Gastroenterol 2014;20(16):4566–73.

58. Uedo N, Iishi H, Tatsuta M, et al. Longterm outcomes after endoscopic mucosal resection for early gastric cancer. Gastric Cancer 2006;9(2):88–92.

59. Kim SG. Endoscopic treatment for early gastric cancer. J Gastric Cancer 2011; 11(3):146–54.

60. Horiki N, Omata F, Uemura M, et al. Risk for local recurrence of early gastric cancer treated with piecemeal endoscopic mucosal resection during a 10-year follow-up period. Surg Endosc 2012;26(1):72–8.

61. Manner H, Rabenstein T, May A, et al. Long-term results of endoscopic resection in early gastric cancer: the western experience. Am J Gastroenterol 2009; 104(3):566–73.

62. Nagano H, Ohyama S, Fukunaga T, et al. Indications for gastrectomy after incomplete EMR for early gastric cancer. Gastric Cancer 2005;8(3):149–54.

63. Facciorusso A, Antonino M, Di Maso M, et al. Endoscopic submucosal dissection vs endoscopic mucosal resection for early gastric cancer: a meta-analysis. World J Gastrointest Endosc 2014;6(11):555–63.

64. Gambitta P, Iannuzzi F, Ballerini A, et al. Endoscopic submucosal dissection versus endoscopic mucosal resection for type 0-II superficial gastric lesions larger than 20 mm. Ann Gastroenterol 2018;31(3):338–43.

65. Cho J-H, Cha S-W, Kim HG, et al. Long-term outcomes of endoscopic submucosal dissection for early gastric cancer: a comparison study to surgery using propensity score-matched analysis. Surg Endosc 2016;30(9):3762–73.

66. Lee S, Choi KD, Han M, et al. Long-term outcomes of endoscopic submucosal dissection versus surgery in early gastric cancer meeting expanded indication including undifferentiated-type tumors: a criteria-based analysis. Gastric Cancer 2018;21(3):490–9.

67. Abdelfatah MM, Barakat M, Lee H, et al. The incidence of lymph node metastasis in early gastric cancer according to the expanded criteria in comparison with the absolute criteria of the Japanese Gastric Cancer Association: a systematic review of the literature and meta-analysis. Gastrointest Endosc 2018;87(2): 338–47.

68. Hiki N, Nunobe S, Kubota T, et al. Function-preserving gastrectomy for early gastric cancer. Ann Surg Oncol 2013;20(8):2683–92.

69. Saito T, Kurokawa Y, Takiguchi S, et al. Current status of function-preserving surgery for gastric cancer. World J Gastroenterol 2014;20(46):17297–304.

70. Oh S-Y, Lee H-J, Yang H-K. Pylorus-preserving gastrectomy for gastric cancer. J Gastric Cancer 2016;16(2):63–71.

71. Park DJ, Lee H-J, Jung HC, et al. Clinical outcome of pylorus-preserving gastrectomy in gastric cancer in comparison with conventional distal gastrectomy with Billroth I anastomosis. World J Surg 2008;32(6):1029–36.

72. Iseki J, Takagi M, Touyama K, et al. Feasibility of central gastrectomy for gastric cancer. Surgery 2003;133(1):68–73.

73. Karanicolas PJ, Graham D, Gönen M, et al. Quality of life after gastrectomy for adenocarcinoma: a prospective cohort study. Ann Surg 2013;257(6):1039–46.

74. Kinami S, Funaki H, Fujita H, et al. Local resection of the stomach for gastric cancer. Surg Today 2017;47(6):651–9.

75. Folkert I, Roses R. Endoscopic full-thickness resection with laparoscopic assistance. Tech Gastrointest Endosc 2015;17(3):112–4.

76. Niimi K, Ishibashi R, Mitsui T, et al. Laparoscopic and endoscopic cooperative surgery for gastrointestinal tumor. Ann Transl Med 2017;5(8). Available at: https://www.ncbi.nlm.nih.gov/pmc/articles/PMC5464944/.

77. Hiki N, Nunobe S, Matsuda T, et al. Laparoscopic endoscopic cooperative surgery. Dig Endosc 2015;27(2):197–204.

78. Tsujimoto H, Yaguchi Y, Kumano I, et al. Successful gastric submucosal tumor resection using laparoscopic and endoscopic cooperative surgery. World J Surg 2012;36(2):327–30.

79. Kitagawa Y, Takeuchi H. Sentinel node navigation surgery for early gastric cancer. In: Morita SY, Balch CM, Klimberg VS, et al, editors. Textbook of complex general

surgical oncology. New York: McGraw-Hill Education; 2018. p. 1001–4. Available at: accesssurgery.mhmedical.com/content.aspx?aid=1145761515.

80. Miyashiro I, Hiratsuka M, Sasako M, et al. High false-negative proportion of intra-operative histological examination as a serious problem for clinical application of sentinel node biopsy for early gastric cancer: final results of the Japan Clinical Oncology Group multicenter trial JCOG0302. Gastric Cancer 2014;17(2): 316–23.

81. Kitamura T, Tanabe S, Koizumi W, et al. Argon plasma coagulation for early gastric cancer: technique and outcome. Gastrointest Endosc 2006;63(1):48–54.

82. Ginsberg GG. The art and science of painting in early gastric cancer: is there a role for ablation therapy? Gastrointest Endosc 2006;63(1):55–9.

83. van der Post RS, Vogelaar IP, Carneiro F, et al. Hereditary diffuse gastric cancer: updated clinical guidelines with an emphasis on germline CDH1 mutation carriers. J Med Genet 2015;52(6):361–74.

84. Schieman C, Wigle DA, Deschamps C, et al. Patterns of operative mortality following esophagectomy. Dis Esophagus 2012;25(7):645–51.

85. Hulscher JBF, van Sandick JW, de Boer AGEM, et al. Extended transthoracic resection compared with limited transhiatal resection for adenocarcinoma of the esophagus. N Engl J Med 2002;347(21):1662–9.

86. Chu KM, Law SY, Fok M, et al. A prospective randomized comparison of transhiatal and transthoracic resection for lower-third esophageal carcinoma. Am J Surg 1997;174(3):320–4.

87. Goldminc M, Maddern G, Le Prise E, et al. Oesophagectomy by a transhiatal approach or thoracotomy: a prospective randomized trial. Br J Surg 1993; 80(3):367–70.

88. Lin J, Iannettoni MD. Transhiatal esophagectomy. Surg Clin North Am 2005; 85(3):593–610.

89. Pennathur A, Gibson MK, Jobe BA, et al. Oesophageal carcinoma. Lancet 2013; 381(9864):400–12.

90. Luketich JD, Pennathur A, Awais O, et al. Outcomes after minimally invasive esophagectomy. Ann Surg 2012;256(1):95–103.

91. Zeng J, Liu J-S. Quality of life after three kinds of esophagectomy for cancer. World J Gastroenterol 2012;18(36):5106–13.

92. Omloo JMT, Lagarde SM, Hulscher JBF, et al. Extended transthoracic resection compared with limited transhiatal resection for adenocarcinoma of the mid/distal esophagus: five-year survival of a randomized clinical trial. Ann Surg 2007; 246(6):992–1000 [discussion: 1000–1].

93. Lazzarino AI, Nagpal K, Bottle A, et al. Open versus minimally invasive esophagectomy: trends of utilization and associated outcomes in England. Ann Surg 2010;252(2):292–8.

94. Yerokun BA, Sun Z, Yang C-FJ, et al. Minimally invasive versus open esophagectomy for esophageal cancer: a population-based analysis. Ann Thorac Surg 2016;102(2):416–23.

95. Tapias LF, Mathisen DJ, Wright CD, et al. Outcomes with open and minimally invasive ivor lewis esophagectomy after neoadjuvant therapy. Ann Thorac Surg 2016;101(3):1097–103.

96. Dunbar KB, Spechler SJ. The risk of lymph-node metastases in patients with high-grade dysplasia or intramucosal carcinoma in Barrett's esophagus: a systematic review. Am J Gastroenterol 2012;107(6):850–62 [quiz: 863].

97. D'Journo XB, Thomas PA. Current management of esophageal cancer. J Thorac Dis 2014;6(Suppl 2):S253–64.

98. Pech O, Behrens A, May A, et al. Long-term results and risk factor analysis for recurrence after curative endoscopic therapy in 349 patients with high-grade intraepithelial neoplasia and mucosal adenocarcinoma in Barrett's oesophagus. Gut 2008;57(9):1200–6.

99. Prasad GA, Wu TT, Wigle DA, et al. Endoscopic and surgical treatment of mucosal (T1a) esophageal adenocarcinoma in Barrett's esophagus. Gastroenterology 2009;137(3):815–23.

100. Chennat J, Konda VJA, Ross AS, et al. Complete Barrett's eradication endoscopic mucosal resection: an effective treatment modality for high-grade dysplasia and intramucosal carcinoma–an American single-center experience. Am J Gastroenterol 2009;104(11):2684–92.

101. Newton AD, Predina JD, Xia L, et al. Surgical management of early-stage esophageal adenocarcinoma based on lymph node metastasis risk. Ann Surg Oncol 2018;25(1):318–25.

102. Merkow RP, Bilimoria KY, Keswani RN, et al. Treatment trends, risk of lymph node metastasis, and outcomes for localized esophageal cancer. J Natl Cancer Inst 2014;106(7) [pii:dju133].

103. Ballard DD, Choksi N, Lin J, et al. Outcomes of submucosal (T1b) esophageal adenocarcinomas removed by endoscopic mucosal resection. World J Gastrointest Endosc 2016;8(20):763–9.

104. Ono S, Fujishiro M, Niimi K, et al. Long-term outcomes of endoscopic submucosal dissection for superficial esophageal squamous cell neoplasms. Gastrointest Endosc 2009;70(5):860–6.

105. Sun F, Yuan P, Chen T, et al. Efficacy and complication of endoscopic submucosal dissection for superficial esophageal carcinoma: a systematic review and meta-analysis. J Cardiothorac Surg 2014;9:78.

106. Yamada M, Oda I, Nonaka S, et al. Long-term outcome of endoscopic resection of superficial adenocarcinoma of the esophagogastric junction. Endoscopy 2013;45(12):992–6.

107. Mocanu A, Bârla R, Hoara P, et al. Current endoscopic methods of radical therapy in early esophageal cancer. J Med Life 2015;8(2):150–6.

108. Buttar NS, Wang KK, Lutzke LS, et al. Combined endoscopic mucosal resection and photodynamic therapy for esophageal neoplasia within Barrett's esophagus. Gastrointest Endosc 2001;54(6):682–8.

109. Pacifico RJ, Wang KK, Wongkeesong LM, et al. Combined endoscopic mucosal resection and photodynamic therapy versus esophagectomy for management of early adenocarcinoma in Barrett's esophagus. Clin Gastroenterol Hepatol 2003; 1(4):252–7. Available at: https://www.cghjournal.org/article/S1542-3565(03)00129-0/fulltext. Accessed August 12, 2018.

110. Milashka M, Calomme A, Van Laethem JL, et al. Sixteen-year follow-up of Barrett's esophagus, endoscopically treated with argon plasma coagulation. United European Gastroenterol J 2014;2(5):367–73.

111. Kim HP, Bulsiewicz WJ, Cotton CC, et al. Focal endoscopic mucosal resection before radiofrequency ablation is equally effective and safe compared with radiofrequency ablation alone for the eradication of Barrett's esophagus with advanced neoplasia. Gastrointest Endosc 2012;76(4):733–9.

What Is the Best Operation for Proximal Gastric Cancer and Distal Esophageal Cancer?

Laura M. Mazer, MD, MS[a], George A. Poultsides, MD, MS[b],*

KEYWORDS

- Gastroesophageal junction • Gastric cancer • Esophageal cancer • Siewert
- Gastrectomy • Esophagectomy

KEY POINTS

- Cancer of the gastroesophageal junction (GEJ) is increasing in frequency.
- Treatment for GEJ tumors is controversial, in part because defining and classifying these lesions is difficult.
- Siewert class I tumors should be treated with either transthoracic or transhiatal esophagectomy. The former approach is associated with a more extensive and precise mediastinal nodal dissection at the expense of increased morbidity; however, both approaches have equivalent long-term survival.
- Siewert II tumors can metastasize to both abdominal and mediastinal lymph nodes, so the resection strategy (esophagectomy or total gastrectomy with resection of the distal esophagus) should involve dissection of paracardial, lesser curvature, left gastric and lower thoracic para-esophageal nodes.
- Siewert III tumors can be treated with either proximal or total gastrectomy. Total gastrectomy provides higher lymph node counts and lower rates of anastomotic stricture and reflux esophagitis.

INTRODUCTION

The incidence of gastric cancer has been decreasing in the western world since the 1970s. The incidence of proximal gastric cancer, however, is rising, along with distal esophageal cancer (primarily adenocarcinoma), and cancer of the gastroesophageal junction (GEJ).[1] These trends are expected to continue in the next decades,[2] likely due to the availability of treatment for *Helicobacter pylori*, as well as increasing rates of obesity and gastroesophageal reflux disease (GERD).[3] For all of these reasons,

[a] Division of Minimally Invasive Surgery, Cedars-Sinai Medical Center, 8635 W. Third Street, West Medical Office Tower, Suite 795, Los Angeles, CA 90048, USA; [b] Section of Surgical Oncology, Stanford University School of Medicine, Stanford University Hospital, 300 pasteur drive, H3680, Stanford, CA 94305, USA
* Corresponding author.
E-mail address: gpoultsides@stanford.edu

Surg Clin N Am 99 (2019) 457–469
https://doi.org/10.1016/j.suc.2019.02.003
0039-6109/19/© 2019 Elsevier Inc. All rights reserved.

surgical.theclinics.com

there is increasing interest in cancers that arise in the space between the esophagus and the stomach: the GEJ.

THE GASTROESOPHAGEAL JUNCTION: AN ANATOMIC ENIGMA

The border between the esophagus and the stomach has been defined based on endoscopic, pathologic, physiologic, and histologic features. Each of these definitions (**Table 1**) has strengths and challenges. Functionally, the stomach stores and digests food, by closing off the lumen proximally at the lower esophageal sphincter (LES) and distally at the pylorus. From a functional standpoint, the most distal end of the LES is the edge of the stomach.[4] This boundary can only be established by manometry, however, making it a challenging practical definition.

Histologically, the squamous cell mucosa of the esophagus is separated from the columnar cell mucosa of the stomach by a small area of "junctional mucosa," composed of mucus-secreting glands in the true gastric cardia.[4–6] Some pathologists argue that this area of unique mucosa is not a true anatomic finding, but rather the result of metaplastic changes in the face of GERD.[7] Evidence to support the existence of a histologically distinct region comes from biopsy studies in pediatric populations, where children without any evidence of reflux are found to have gastric cardiac glands.[5] This supports the existence of a small region unique in cell type and function from either the esophagus or the stomach.

The most common definition, because it is the most practical to apply, is the anatomic/endoscopic location of the GEJ. Even here, however, there are controversies. On endoscopy, the squamocolumnar junction is commonly used as a landmark for the GEJ, although its location is easily obscured by inflammation.[4] In Europe and the United States, the most common anatomic definition is the extreme proximal end of the gastric folds.[8] The gastric folds can be obscured as well, by inflating the stomach with air, the presence of gastric mucosal atrophy, or a large proximal gastric mass. In Japan, the GEJ is commonly defined as the distal end of the lower esophageal palisade vessels, which can be seen endoscopically as well as on pathology, allowing for preoperative classification and postoperative confirmation of tumor location with relation to the GEJ.[4]

The GEJ remains an area of controversy today. It is a space of centimeters with a function, histology, and anatomy unique from either the esophagus or the stomach. But the exact location of the region is hard to define, and this uncertainty is relevant to surgeons. This article discusses the challenges in determining optimal surgical resection for GEJ cancer, using a classification schema that divides the already-contentious location of the GEJ into even smaller subdivisions. Understanding the challenges in defining the GEJ is important to interpreting and applying data on the best surgical strategy for tumors arising in this unique space.

Table 1	
Definitions of the gastroesophageal junction (GEJ)	
Function	The Distal End of the LES, Defined by Manometry
Histology	The area of junctional mucosa containing cardiac glands that separate the squamous mucosa of the distal esophagus from the columnar mucosa of the fundus of the stomach
Anatomy	Squamocolumnar junction seen on endoscopy Most proximal end of the gastric folds Incisura (angle of His) Edge of the lower esophageal palisade vessels

Abbreviation: LES, lower esophageal sphincter.

CLASSIFYING GASTROESOPHAGEAL JUNCTION CANCER: SIEWERT AND TUMOR-NODES-METASTASIS

Not surprisingly given the confusion regarding the anatomic and histologic definition of the GEJ, clinicians have struggled with classification of tumors arising in this area. These tumors have been considered by some to be esophageal carcinomas, by some to be gastric, and by others to represent a separate third entity altogether. Since the 1980s, the Siewert classification system has been used in an attempt to standardize diagnosis, reporting, and research on these tumors.[9-12] In Siewert's initial papers, the GEJ was defined as the most proximal end of the gastric folds, and he identifies 3 types of tumors based on where the lesion arises (**Fig. 1**):[13]

- Siewert type I: adenocarcinoma of the distal esophagus, infiltrating the GEJ from above

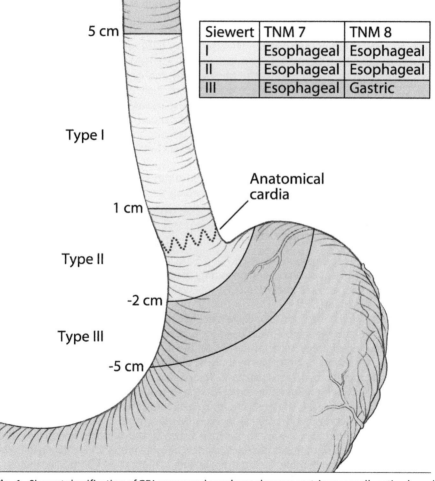

Siewert	TNM 7	TNM 8
I	Esophageal	Esophageal
II	Esophageal	Esophageal
III	Esophageal	Gastric

Fig. 1. Siewert classification of GEJ cancer and esophageal versus gastric cancer allocation based on the seventh and eighth editions of the AJCC TNM staging system. Data in Table from Rice TW, Blackstone EH, Rusch VW. 7th edition of the AJCC Cancer Staging Manual: esophagus and esophagogastric junction. Ann Surg Oncol 2010;17: 1721–4 and Rice TW, Patil DT, Blackstone EH. 8th edition AJCC/UICC staging of cancers of the esophagus and esophagogastric junction: application to clinical practice. Ann Cardiothorac Surg 2017;6:119–30.

- Siewert type II: true carcinoma of the cardia, arising from the cardiac epithelium at the GEJ
- Siewert type III: subcardia gastric carcinoma, which infiltrates the GEJ from below

The Siewert classification provides a unifying framework for discussing GEJ tumors, and was selected as the consensus standard for defining, assessing, and reporting GEJ cancers by the International Gastric Cancer Association in 2000.[12] Siewert I often arises in the setting of Barrett esophagus, similar to distal esophageal cancer. Siewert III, in contrast, often shares features of gastric cancer, including *H pylori* infection, gastritis, and eosinophilia.[14]

The Siewert classification provides a valuable tool to discuss management and plan surgical resection, but it is not without limitations. It does not consider tumor biology or genetics. It also relies on a clearly defined GEJ, to confidently classify a tumor as arising a centimeter above, or 2 below, the true GEJ, and does not make allowances for tumors that straddle 2 Siewert classifications. Pathologic determination of Siewert classification matches preoperative endoscopic determination in only 64% to 72%, and preoperative radiographic determination in only 57% to 72%.[15–17]

The American Joint Commission on Cancer (AJCC) TNM Classification of GEJ tumors differs slightly from Siewert, and has recently changed. The eighth edition defines GEJ tumors based on their epicenter, rather than their upper edge, as was done in the seventh edition. The eighth addition also reclassifies the GEJ: previously, all cancers of the GEJ were staged as esophageal cancer.[18] In the eighth edition, adenocarcinomas with epicenters no more than 2 cm into the gastric cardia (Siewert I and II) are considered esophageal cancer, and tumors farther than 2 cm into the cardia (Siewert III) are staged as gastric cancer.[19]

A discussion of the surgical options for GEJ tumors must be placed within the context of the controversy and confusion regarding the nature of the GEJ itself, and the imperfect ways in which tumors arising in this region are classified.

SURGICAL RESECTION: SIEWERT CLASS I

Siewert class I tumors, located between 1 and 5 cm from the GEJ, are the least controversial to manage. In all classification schemata these are considered true esophageal adenocarcinomas, and are treated accordingly with esophagectomy and mediastinal lymph node dissection.[20,21]

The 2 most popular methods to achieve resection of a distal esophageal cancer differ according to whether thoracotomy is used for esophageal mobilization. *Transthoracic esophagectomy* performed through a right thoracotomy and laparotomy (Ivor Lewis or Tanner-Lewis esophagectomy) allow for lymphadenectomy to be performed sharply in both fields (abdomen and mediastinum). The gastric conduit is brought through the posterior mediastinum and the anastomosis is performed in the chest at or above the level of the azygous vein. Alternatively, the anastomosis can be performed in the neck through a separate left cervical incision (McKeown or 3-field approach). The thoracic anastomosis has a lower leak rate than a cervical anastomosis, but on the other hand, intrathoracic anastomoses are hampered by a higher reoperation rate when there is a postoperative anastomotic leak (approximately 4% to 10%).[22] The thoracotomy approach overall carries higher peri-procedural morbidity and mortality.[23,24]

Transhiatal esophagectomy is performed with blunt mobilization of the intrathoracic esophagus from the esophageal hiatus and from a left cervical incision to the thoracic inlet without the need for thoracotomy. The advantage of the transhiatal technique is that it avoids thoracotomy while achieving a complete removal of the esophagus. The potential disadvantages include a limited periesophageal and mediastinal lymphade-nectomy, and the risk of causing tracheobronchial or vascular injury during blunt dissection of the esophagus (especially for locally advanced tumors). A cervical anas-tomosis is associated with a higher rate of anastomotic leakage than an intrathoracic anastomosis (12% vs 5%, respectively), although the morbidity of a thoracic leak is much higher.[22] Other potential downsides to a cervical anastomosis include pharyn-geal reflux, nocturnal aspiration, and prolonged swallowing dysfunction and hoarse-ness after surgery, due to an increased incidence of recurrent laryngeal nerve palsy.[25] This last complication is underestimated in its importance: a patient with an intrathoracic stomach and limited ability to protect his or her airway is at great danger in the immediate postoperative period and is also in chronic danger of aspiration.

Great controversy remains over the value and extent of lymphadenectomy. There is one group of thought that lymph node metastases are markers for systemic disease and that removal of involved nodes in most cases offers no survival benefit. This is very likely to be true when more than 8 lymph nodes are involved with cancer on the sur-gical specimen.[26] However, many well-respected and experienced surgeons believe that some patients with affected lymph nodes can achieve a durable survival or even cure with an aggressive surgical approach that focuses on wide peritumoral excision and extended lymphadenectomy using a transthoracic/thoracoabdominal approach (en bloc or radical esophagectomy).[27] There is currently no definitive evidence to sup-port either philosophy; however, in specific subsets of T3N1 patients, complete lympha-denectomy provides prolonged survival and excellent locoregional control in comparison with transhiatal resection.[28] It is unclear whether more extensive dissection actually leads to improved survival through improved locoregional control or whether these superior results are a function of more accurate staging (stage migration effect). Prospective randomized studies in Western Europe have failed to show any significant difference in recurrence-free or overall survival rate when comparing transhiatal with transthoracic esophagectomy.[29] Because an overall survival benefit has yet to be proven, either technique is acceptable. The choice among surgical resection techniques should be individualized to the particular characteristics of the patient. Subset analyses have shown that in the presence of limited lymph node involvement (1–8 positive nodes), a complete (at least 2 fields, including a thoracic dissection) esophagectomy can be associated with a survival benefit compared with a transhiatal resection.[28,30] The salient points that emerge from historical comparisons of these procedures is that a transhiatal resection has a tendency toward higher locoregional recurrence, but a lower incidence of intensive care unit care, and does not require thoracotomy to complete. We person-ally advocate for a transthoracic approach to resection of distal esophageal cancers, but reserve a transhiatal approach for patients who due to age or comorbidities are at high risk for thoracotomy.

Minimally invasive esophagogastrectomy is offered in many centers around the world. Patients with appropriate lesions have the option of undergoing esophageal resection with combined thoracoscopic and laparoscopic resection with the esopha-gogastric anastomosis performed in the chest or in the neck. Complete laparoscopic (transhiatal) resections can also be accomplished, but again, this approach makes extensive en bloc resection of mediastinal lymph nodes difficult. Early results on several hundred patients resected in this manner show no difference in survival, and a formal phase III trial is currently under way.[31] Disadvantages of this modality include a fairly steep learning curve, especially for surgeons with limited laparoscopic esoph-ageal experience and prolonged anesthetic times (although surgeons with extensive experience in minimally invasive techniques can effectively resect the esophagus in a similar amount of time as open procedures).

SURGICAL RESECTION: SIEWERT CLASS II

Siewert class II tumors arise in the true gastric cardia and are, perhaps, the most difficult to define and treat. Options for surgical resection include total gastrectomy with distal esophagectomy (through an abdominal/transhiatal or left thoracoabdominal approach) and esophagectomy (through a transhiatal or transthoracic approach as described for Siewert I tumors). No true consensus exists, in part because very few randomized controlled trials have treated the GEJ as its own unique zone.[20]

Resection margin status and length may impact survival, and technical considerations regarding proximal margin can impact choice of resection strategy. The most important prognostic factor for survival remains an R0 resection, regardless of tumor type or operative approach.[32] Longer resection margins decrease the likelihood of microscopically positive margins. In a retrospective analysis of patients with Siewert II and III cancer, Ito and colleagues[33] found a 35% rate of R1 resection because of a positive proximal margin, but no incidence of microscopic disease if the macroscopic resection margin length was $\geq$6 cm. Barbour and colleagues[34] in 2007 found that patients with a negative margin greater than 3.8 cm ex vivo (or 5 cm in situ) had significantly better survival than those with shorter margins, even when controlling for stage. Not surprisingly, patients treated with extended gastrectomy had significantly shorter proximal margins than those treated with esophagectomy (1.75 cm vs 4 cm). However, a more recent retrospective cohort study in Sweden found no difference in negative margin rates between total gastrectomy and esophagectomy,[35] and a study by the US Gastric Cancer Collaborative demonstrated no relationship between proximal margin length and local recurrence or survival.[36] Putting these data together, it appears that esophagectomy may provide a longer proximal resection margin for type II GEJ tumors; however, both approaches (gastrectomy and esophagectomy) appear to offer similar rates of margin-negative resections and obtaining a specific proximal margin length is not sufficient justification for routine esophagectomy.

Lymph node dissection is another major goal of surgical resection. The presence of lymph node metastases is a strong adverse predictor of survival,[30] although the ideal number or location for lymph node sampling in GEJ tumors is under debate. AJCC considers 15 lymph nodes adequate staging for gastric cancer, but this number is less well defined for esophageal cancer, with numbers ranging from 10 to 40.[37,38] Administrative database studies suggest that the number of lymph nodes resected may be a prognostic factor in GEJ cancer, with 21 or more nodes indicating better survival.[37] Like all studies of this kind, this conclusion is limited due to lack of data on chemotherapy, pathologic margin status, and standardized protocols for either dissection or pathologic evaluation of nodes.

Studies and guidelines focusing on the number of resected lymph nodes do not necessarily include information regarding location of the nodal basin to be dissected. The GEJ has lymphatic drainage pathways to both mediastinal and abdominal fields (**Fig. 2**). Leers and colleagues[39] showed that for patients with N1 disease, more than 40% had involved nodes in the mediastinum, and in 8% of patients, the only positive nodes were in the chest. Other groups have looked at the specific therapeutic contribution that dissection of each specific nodal station has to offer. Yamashita and colleagues[40] found that the highest therapeutic benefit for GEJ cancer was in taking the paracardial and lesser curvature nodes, with less benefit for greater curvature and parapyloric node harvest, although they combined both Siewert II and III types. Hasegawa and colleagues[21] looked at each Siewert subtype separately: they found for all patients that the paracardial and lesser curvature nodes (stations 1, 2, and 3)

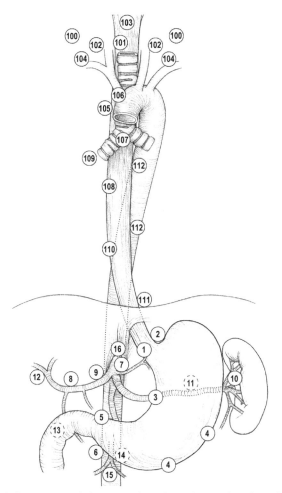

Fig. 2. Lymph node basins around the stomach and esophagus that drain the GEJ, based on guidelines. (*From* the Japanese Society for Esophageal Diseases: guidelines for the clinical and pathologic studies for carcinoma of the esophagus. Jpn J Surg 1976;6:70; with permission.)

were the most beneficial, followed by nodes at the root of the left gastric artery (station 7). After that, in Siewert II tumors, the next highest therapeutic value index is in resection of lower thoracic para-esophageal nodes (station 110). However, it is debatable whether a thoracotomy is necessary for this lower mediastinal lymph node dissection. Sasako and colleagues[41] started a multicenter, prospective randomized phase III trial for patients with GEJ and cardia gastric cancer comparing abdominal transhiatal total gastrectomy with total gastrectomy through a left thoracoabdominal approach (which included a thorough mediastinal lymphadenectomy below the left inferior pulmonary vein). The trial was closed prematurely, as at interim analysis there was increased morbidity with the left thoracoabdominal approach, without any associated survival benefit.[42]

Long-term quality of life and survival also play very important roles in determining the ideal resection strategy: a meta-analysis of 10 observational cohort studies (7 retrospective and 3 prospective, including the landmark article by Rudiger Siewert and colleagues[12]) showed that neither esophagectomy, nor gastrectomy offered an apparent 5-year survival benefit, as R0 resection rates and lymph node yields were similar. Morbidity and mortality rates were also comparable for both techniques, but long-term quality of life was more severely affected after esophagectomy than gastrectomy, including global quality of life outcomes, function role (work and leisure), social function, and fatigue.[23] Similarly, Siewert and colleagues[32] in their original series of more than 1000 patients found no differences in survival between patients undergoing total gastrectomy with transhiatal resection of the distal esophagus, and those undergoing complete abdominothoracic esophagectomy with proximal gastrectomy and 2-field lymphadenectomy.

As mentioned previously, comparing transhiatal and transthoracic esophagectomy, several studies including 2 recent meta-analyses have failed to show any survival difference between the 2 techniques.[25,30,43]

For true carcinomas of the GEJ (Siewert II tumors), both total gastrectomy (with transhiatal distal esophagectomy) and esophagectomy (transthoracic or transhiatal) are entirely acceptable strategies. Tumor characteristics should guide the choice of approach: for tumors that extend more into the stomach, a total gastrectomy may be more appropriate; for tumors extending more into the esophagus, an esophagectomy may provide a more comfortable proximal margin. If the tumor is confined to the GEJ, surgeon experience should guide the selection of approach. A total gastrectomy with distal esophagectomy through a left thoracoabdominal exposure may facilitate achieving a negative proximal margin for bulky cardia/fundus tumors invading high up in the distal thoracic esophagus, but should be used selectively only in these circumstances, due to increased morbidity.

SURGICAL RESECTION: SIEWERT CLASS III

Siewert class III tumors represent almost half of all GEJ cancers, and carry the worst prognosis.[44] They were initially classified as esophageal cancer in the seventh TNM edition, and were reclassified as gastric cancer in the eighth edition (see **Fig. 1**). Surgical goals remain an R0 resection, with appropriate lymph node clearance, while minimizing procedural morbidity. However, like the other 2 Siewert types, there is debate regarding the ideal operation to achieve those aims. Overall, Siewert type III cancers are now defined as gastric cancer invading the esophagus, and surgical options include proximal gastrectomy (PG) and total gastrectomy (TG).

Traditionally, these tumors were treated with complete gastric resection based on a landmark study by Papachristou and Fortner[45] in 1980. Their retrospective analysis of 101 patients showed longer negative margins, higher lymph node harvests, and lower local recurrence rates, although not better overall survival, with TG versus PG. TG carries significant morbidity, however, including postoperative anemia (due to iron and B12 malabsorption), weight loss, and failure to thrive, and some investigators propose that PG may be able to provide a better quality of life without sacrificing oncologic outcomes.[46,47] PG can retain part of the gastric reservoir, vagal input and hormone secretion, and preserves the pylorus, leading proponents to argue that retaining some stomach will lead to better functional outcomes.[46]

Resection margin length is a matter of debate for Siewert type III, as they are in type II. There are studies indicating that a resection margin greater than 2 cm[48] or even 5 cm[34] may improve overall survival. Overall, most studies recommend a margin of 4 to 6 cm for all Siewert types.[44] As with Siewert II, however, there remains uncertainty, and a shorter length of negative margin may be acceptable.[36]

Lymph node dissection for type III tumors are similar to type II; the nodal basins with the highest therapeutic value (calculated based on both likelihood of metastatic disease, and survival impact from dissection of this basin) are still the paracardial and lesser curve nodes (stations 1, 2, and 3), followed by station 7 at the root of the left gastric artery.[21] After that, however, the most important basins differed between type II and III tumors, with the lower thoracic para-esophageal nodes (basin 110) being important for type II, and the nodes along the splenic artery and splenic hilum (10 and 11p) more useful in type III. Furthermore, the incidence of metastasis in the suprapyloric and infrapyloric nodes (stations 5 and 6) is approximately 10% in patients with proximal gastric cancer of advanced T stage, and these positive nodes would be left in situ after a PG, leading to an incomplete resection.[49] In general, the AJCC defines a minimum of 15 lymph nodes examined as adequate for a gastric cancer resection, and in the eighth TNM staging this would also apply to Siewert III tumors. There is evidence to suggest that higher lymph node counts (of 25 or even 35) may improve survival after resection of gastric cancer,[50,51] although this has not been evaluated specifically for GEJ tumors.

Although the importance of margin length, and extent of lymph node dissection are not unequivocally proven, TG does provide larger margins and a greater lymph node harvest than PG, maintaining a similar *perioperative morbidity* profile.[47,52,53] However, this difference has not been translated into a *survival* advantage.[45]

Therefore, some investigators argue that one should perform a PG for Siewert III adenocarcinoma of the GEJ, noting that TG does not improve prognosis. However, some studies have shown that PG actually carries a worse *quality of life* (primarily due to reflux) than TG. Long-term complications from either operation are primarily anastomotic stricture or reflux esophagitis, with conflicting results in the literature regarding which approach is superior. Some groups showed higher rates of stricture and esophagitis with TG[53]; some showed a higher rate of both complications with PG[47]; and others showed no difference.[54] Two large meta-analyses of 3 randomized clinical trials and 9 retrospective studies, however, found overall significantly higher rates of reflux esophagitis and anastomotic stricture after PG compared with TG.[55,56] Patient-reported quality of life outcomes are mixed. PG is associated in some studies with reduced dumping and less need for additional meals.[57] Other studies have shown a decreased quality of life with PG, due to higher rates of clinically significant reflux and nausea.[58] Importantly, the reconstruction methods after PG or TG are not standardized, and many studies compare patients with different reconstruction methods, including Roux-en-y reconstruction (with or without jejunal pouch), Billroth II, gastric pull-up, and jejunal interposition grafts.[52,59]

At the authors' institution, we usually perform a TG with a Roux-en-Y reconstruction and regional lymphadenectomy for proximal gastric cancer. This procedure has the advantage of avoiding the alkaline reflux esophagitis often associated with PG. Furthermore, lymph nodes along the lesser curvature, a common site of spread, are easily removed during TG with similar rates of mortality or morbidity compared with PG.

SUMMARY

Despite advancements in chemotherapy and radiotherapy, surgical resection remains the mainstay of treatment for cancer of the GEJ. The goals of surgical therapy are those of any gastrointestinal cancer operation: obtaining an R0 resection with adequate lymph node dissection, minimizing perioperative morbidity and mortality, while maximizing survival and long-term quality of life.

Classification and treatment of GEJ tumors remains challenging, and the available data have significant limitations. The GEJ itself is a point of controversy, and it is defined variably by different disciplines. The recent change in classification of Siewert III GEJ cancers as gastric, rather than esophageal, in the new AJCC 8 staging system highlights the confusion regarding the nature of these lesions. The Siewert system, the most commonly used and the most beneficial for standardizing research and diagnosis, still mischaracterizes up to 30% of tumors preoperatively. To increase confusion, many studies still combine 2 or even all 3 of Siewert subgroups, contributing to the lack of clarity in describing the implications of resection. Finally, there is little standardization in the available literature regarding the type of neoadjuvant or adjuvant multimodal therapy, or technique of reconstruction after resection.

When deciding on the optimal surgical strategy for distal esophageal and proximal gastric cancer, an appreciation for the limits of the currently available literature is important. That being said, some generalizable conclusions can be drawn. Siewert type I tumors are best treated with esophagectomy, and there are no data to clearly support a transthoracic over transhiatal approach. The former approach is associated with a more extensive mediastinal nodal dissection (and perhaps improved locoregional control) at the expense of increased morbidity. However, both approaches are equivalent in terms of long-term outcomes. Siewert type II tumors are perhaps the most controversial in terms of optimal resection strategy; however, it is clear that they can metastasize to both lower mediastinal/peri-esophageal and abdominal lymph nodes. Whether a TG (with transhiatal distal esophagectomy) or an esophagectomy (transthoracic or transhiatal) is chosen, it should provide dissection of lymph node stations 1, 2, 3, 7, and 110, as well as adequate negative margins. For Siewert type III tumors, proximal and TG may provide equivalent oncologic outcomes, although TG is preferable as it carries a lower risk of anastomotic stricture and reflux esophagitis.

REFERENCES

1. Buas MF, Vaughan TL. Epidemiology and risk factors for gastroesophageal junction tumors: understanding the rising incidence of this disease. Semin Radiat Oncol 2013;23:3–9.
2. Arnold M, Laversanne M, Brown LM, et al. Predicting the future burden of esophageal cancer by histological subtype: international trends in incidence up to 2030. Am J Gastroenterol 2017;112:1247–55.
3. Hashimoto T, Kurokawa Y, Mori M, et al. Surgical treatment of gastroesophageal junction cancer. J Gastric Cancer 2018;18:209–17.
4. Ichihara S, Uedo N, Gotoda T. Considering the esophagogastric junction as a 'zone'. Dig Endosc 2017;29(Suppl 2):3–10.
5. Kilgore SP, Ormsby AH, Gramlich TL, et al. The gastric cardia: fact or fiction? Am J Gastroenterol 2000;95:921–4.
6. OWEN DA. Stomach. In: Sternberg SS, editor. Histology for pathologists. New York: Raven; 1992. p. 533–45.
7. Oberg S, Peters JH, DeMeester TR, et al. Inflammation and specialized intestinal metaplasia of cardiac mucosa is a manifestation of gastroesophageal reflux disease. Ann Surg 1997;226:522–30 [discussion: 530–2].
8. Chandrasoma PT, Der R, Ma Y, et al. Histology of the gastroesophageal junction: an autopsy study. Am J Surg Pathol 2000;24:402–9.
9. Siewert JR, Holscher AH, Becker K, et al. Cardia cancer: attempt at a therapeutically relevant classification. Chirurg 1987;58:25–32 [in German].

10. Siewert JR, Stein HJ, Sendler A, et al. Surgical resection for cancer of the cardia. Semin Surg Oncol 1999;17:125–31.
11. Feith M, Stein HJ, Siewert JR. Adenocarcinoma of the esophagogastric junction: surgical therapy based on 1602 consecutive resected patients. Surg Oncol Clin N Am 2006;15:751–64.
12. Rudiger Siewert J, Feith M, Werner M, et al. Adenocarcinoma of the esophago-gastric junction: results of surgical therapy based on anatomical/topographic classification in 1,002 consecutive patients. Ann Surg 2000;232:353–61.
13. Siewert JR, Stein HJ, Feith M. Adenocarcinoma of the esophago-gastric junction. Scand J Surg 2006;95:260–9.
14. Odze RD. Unraveling the mystery of the gastroesophageal junction: a patholo-gist's perspective. Am J Gastroenterol 2005;100:1853–67.
15. Grotenhuis BA, Wijnhoven BP, Poley JW, et al. Preoperative assessment of tumor location and station-specific lymph node status in patients with adenocarcinoma of the gastroesophageal junction. World J Surg 2013;37:147–55.
16. Pedrazzani C, Bernini M, Giacopuzzi S, et al. Evaluation of Siewert classification in gastro-esophageal junction adenocarcinoma: what is the role of endoscopic ultrasonography? J Surg Oncol 2005;91:226–31.
17. Parry K, Haverkamp L, Bruijnen RC, et al. Staging of adenocarcinoma of the gastroesophageal junction. Eur J Surg Oncol 2016;42:400–6.
18. Rice TW, Blackstone EH, Rusch VW. 7th edition of the AJCC Cancer Staging Manual: esophagus and esophagogastric junction. Ann Surg Oncol 2010;17: 1721–4.
19. Rice TW, Patil DT, Blackstone EH. 8th edition AJCC/UICC staging of cancers of the esophagus and esophagogastric junction: application to clinical practice. Ann Cardiothorac Surg 2017;6:119–30.
20. Hulscher JB, van Sandick JW, de Boer AG, et al. Extended transthoracic resec-tion compared with limited transhiatal resection for adenocarcinoma of the esophagus. N Engl J Med 2002;347:1662–9.
21. Hasegawa S, Yoshikawa T, Rino Y, et al. Priority of lymph node dissection for Sie-wert type II/III adenocarcinoma of the esophagogastric junction. Ann Surg Oncol 2013;20:4252–9.
22. Orringer MB, Marshall B, Iannettoni MD. Transhiatal esophagectomy: clinical experience and refinements. Ann Surg 1999;230:392–400 [discussion: 400–3].
23. Haverkamp L, Ruurda JP, van Leeuwen MS, et al. Systematic review of the surgi-cal strategies of adenocarcinomas of the gastroesophageal junction. Surg Oncol 2014;23:222–8.
24. Hulscher JB, Tijssen JG, Obertop H, et al. Transthoracic versus transhiatal resec-tion for carcinoma of the esophagus: a meta-analysis. Ann Thorac Surg 2001;72: 306–13.
25. Boshier PR, Anderson O, Hanna GB. Transthoracic versus transhiatal esopha-gectomy for the treatment of esophagogastric cancer: a meta-analysis. Ann Surg 2011;254:894–906.
26. Peyre CG, Hagen JA, DeMeester SR, et al. Predicting systemic disease in pa-tients with esophageal cancer after esophagectomy: a multinational study on the significance of the number of involved lymph nodes. Ann Surg 2008;248: 979–85.
27. Hagen JA, DeMeester SR, Peters JH, et al. Curative resection for esophageal adenocarcinoma: analysis of 100 en bloc esophagectomies. Ann Surg 2001; 234:520–30 [discussion: 530–1].

28. Johansson J, DeMeester TR, Hagen JA, et al. En bloc vs transhiatal esophagectomy for stage T3 N1 adenocarcinoma of the distal esophagus. Arch Surg 2004; 139:627–31 [discussion: 627–31].

29. Goldminc M, Maddern G, Le Prise E, et al. Oesophagectomy by a transhiatal approach or thoracotomy: a prospective randomized trial. Br J Surg 1993;80: 367–70.

30. Omloo JM, Lagarde SM, Hulscher JB, et al. Extended transthoracic resection compared with limited transhiatal resection for adenocarcinoma of the mid/distal esophagus: five-year survival of a randomized clinical trial. Ann Surg 2007;246: 992–1000 [discussion: 1000–1].

31. van der Sluis PC, Ruurda JP, van der Horst S, et al. Robot-assisted minimally invasive thoraco-laparoscopic esophagectomy versus open transthoracic esophagectomy for resectable esophageal cancer, a randomized controlled trial (ROBOT trial). Trials 2012;13:230.

32. von Rahden BH, Stein HJ, Siewert JR. Surgical management of esophagogastric junction tumors. World J Gastroenterol 2006;12:6608–13.

33. Ito H, Clancy TE, Osteen RT, et al. Adenocarcinoma of the gastric cardia: what is the optimal surgical approach? J Am Coll Surg 2004;199:880–6.

34. Barbour AP, Rizk NP, Gonen M, et al. Adenocarcinoma of the gastroesophageal junction: influence of esophageal resection margin and operative approach on outcome. Ann Surg 2007;246:1–8.

35. Kauppila JH, Wahlin K, Lagergren J. Gastrectomy compared to oesophagectomy for Siewert II and III gastro-oesophageal junctional cancer in relation to resection margins, lymphadenectomy and survival. Sci Rep 2017;7:17783.

36. Postlewait LM, Squires MH 3rd, Kooby DA, et al. The importance of the proximal resection margin distance for proximal gastric adenocarcinoma: a multi-institutional study of the US Gastric Cancer Collaborative. J Surg Oncol 2015; 112:203–7.

37. Lai S, Su T, He X, et al. Prognostic value of resected lymph nodes numbers for Siewert II gastroesophageal junction cancer. Oncotarget 2018;9:2797–809.

38. Rizk NP, Ishwaran H, Rice TW, et al. Optimum lymphadenectomy for esophageal cancer. Ann Surg 2010;251:46–50.

39. Leers JM, DeMeester SR, Chan N, et al. Clinical characteristics, biologic behavior, and survival after esophagectomy are similar for adenocarcinoma of the gastroesophageal junction and the distal esophagus. J Thorac Cardiovasc Surg 2009;138:594–602 [discussion: 601–2].

40. Yamashita H, Katai H, Morita S, et al. Optimal extent of lymph node dissection for Siewert type II esophagogastric junction carcinoma. Ann Surg 2011;254:274–80.

41. Sasako M, Sano T, Yamamoto S, et al. Left thoracoabdominal approach versus abdominal-transhiatal approach for gastric cancer of the cardia or subcardia: a randomised controlled trial. Lancet Oncol 2006;7:644–51.

42. Kurokawa Y, Sasako M, Sano T, et al. Ten-year follow-up results of a randomized clinical trial comparing left thoracoabdominal and abdominal transhiatal approaches to total gastrectomy for adenocarcinoma of the oesophagogastric junction or gastric cardia. Br J Surg 2015;102:341–8.

43. Wei MT, Zhang YC, Deng XB, et al. Transthoracic vs transhiatal surgery for cancer of the esophagogastric junction: a meta-analysis. World J Gastroenterol 2014;20: 10183–92.

44. Di Leo A, Zanoni A. Siewert III adenocarcinoma: treatment update. Updates Surg 2017;69:319–25.

45. Papachristou DN, Fortner JG. Adenocarcinoma of the gastric cardia. The choice of gastrectomy. Ann Surg 1980;192:58–64.

46. Nomura E, Okajima K. Function-preserving gastrectomy for gastric cancer in Japan. World J Gastroenterol 2016;22:5888–95.

47. Rosa F, Quero G, Fiorillo C, et al. Total vs proximal gastrectomy for adenocarcinoma of the upper third of the stomach: a propensity-score-matched analysis of a multicenter western experience (On behalf of the Italian Research Group for Gastric Cancer-GIRCG). Gastric Cancer 2018;21(15):845–52.

48. Mine S, Sano T, Hiki N, et al. Proximal margin length with transhiatal gastrectomy for Siewert type II and III adenocarcinomas of the oesophagogastric junction. Br J Surg 2013;100:1050–4.

49. Song W, Liu Y, Ye J, et al. Proximal gastric cancer: lymph node metastatic patterns according to different T stages dictate surgical approach. Chin Med J (Engl) 2014;127:4049–54.

50. Nienhuser H, Schmidt T. Gastric cancer lymph node resection-the more the merrier? Transl Gastroenterol Hepatol 2018;3:1.

51. Gholami S, Janson L, Worhunsky DJ, et al. Number of lymph nodes removed and survival after gastric cancer resection: an analysis from the US gastric cancer collaborative. J Am Coll Surg 2015;221:291–9.

52. Sugoor P, Shah S, Dusane R, et al. Proximal gastrectomy versus total gastrectomy for proximal third gastric cancer: total gastrectomy is not always necessary. Langenbecks Arch Surg 2016;401:687–97.

53. Son MW, Kim YJ, Jeong GA, et al. Long-term outcomes of proximal gastrectomy versus total gastrectomy for upper-third gastric cancer. J Gastric Cancer 2014; 14:246–51.

54. Nozaki I, Hato S, Kobatake T, et al. Long-term outcome after proximal gastrectomy with jejunal interposition for gastric cancer compared with total gastrectomy. World J Surg 2013;37:558–64.

55. Pu YW, Gong W, Wu YY, et al. Proximal gastrectomy versus total gastrectomy for proximal gastric carcinoma. A meta-analysis on postoperative complications, 5-year survival, and recurrence rate. Saudi Med J 2013;34:1223–8.

56. Wen L, Chen XZ, Wu B, et al. Total vs. proximal gastrectomy for proximal gastric cancer: a systematic review and meta-analysis. Hepatogastroenterology 2012; 59:633–40.

57. Takiguchi N, Takahashi M, Ikeda M, et al. Long-term quality-of-life comparison of total gastrectomy and proximal gastrectomy by postgastrectomy syndrome assessment scale (PGSAS-45): a nationwide multi-institutional study. Gastric Cancer 2015;18:407–16.

58. Karanicolas PJ, Graham D, Gonen M, et al. Quality of life after gastrectomy for adenocarcinoma: a prospective cohort study. Ann Surg 2013;257:1039–46.

59. Xiao JW, Liu ZL, Ye PC, et al. Clinical comparison of antrum-preserving double tract reconstruction vs roux-en-Y reconstruction after gastrectomy for Siewert types II and III adenocarcinoma of the esophagogastric junction. World J Gastroenterol 2015;21:9999–10007.

The Difficult Esophageal Conduit

Rajat Kumar, MD, Benjamin Wei, MD*

KEYWORDS

- Difficult esophageal conduit • Alternative conduits • Conduits for esophagectomy

KEY POINTS

- Patients with a history of prior gastric surgery may still be candidates for use of stomach as a conduit.
- The popularity of bariatric surgical procedures will affect availability of conduits.
- Familiarity with alternative conduits and jejunal and colonic interposition is a necessity for the esophageal surgeon.
- Current management of postoperative anastomotic leak continues to improve.

Projections estimate that esophageal cancer incidence will continue to rise.[1] With continued improvements in chemotherapy and radiation regimens, many additional patients will present for surgical intervention. Surgeons continue to enhance techniques with improvements in outcomes and decreased postoperative mortality. There will remain a subset of patients who will pose difficulties intraoperatively. These will include patients who have had prior surgery and other procedures, and patients with conditions that can affect the stomach as a future usable conduit. In these situations, consideration should be raised for the use of alternative conduits, including jejunal and colonic interposition conduits. The esophageal surgeon will be required to be adept at management of intraoperative difficulties with the conduit.

PRIOR SURGERY

Prior gastric surgery does not preclude the stomach from use as a conduit. Patients who have had procedures such as percutaneously or surgically placed gastric feeding tubes and prior antireflux or hiatal hernia surgeries can still be considered for use of gastric conduit after mobilization and evaluation. Ideally the enteral feeding tube that had been created after knowledge of the esophageal disease would have been

The authors have nothing to disclose.
Division of Cardiothoracic Surgery, Department of Surgery, University of Alabama Birmingham Medical Center, Birmingham, AL, USA
* Corresponding author. ZRB 701 1720 2nd Avenue South, Birmingham, AL 35294.
E-mail address: bwei@uab.edu

Surg Clin N Am 99 (2019) 471–478
https://doi.org/10.1016/j.suc.2019.02.009
0039-6109/19/Published by Elsevier Inc.

placed with consideration of possible future conduit creation. Enteral feeding access for esophageal cancer is usually placed as a jejunostomy feeding tube; however, a history of a percutaneously placed gastrostomy has been shown to not preclude safe creation of a gastric conduit.[2] Even placement near the greater curvature does not preclude creation of a gastric conduit. Careful dissection and closure of the gastrostomy (stapled or handsewn 2-layer closure) can allow use for neoesophageal creation.

Prior foregut surgeries, ranging from antireflux procedures to hiatal hernia operations, present a challenge to the creation and subsequent use of a gastric conduit. It has been noted that the stomach can still be used in these cases, but this is associated with increased operative time and increased risk of postoperative complications including anastomotic leak.[3,4] However, during mobilization of the greater curvature of the stomach during a fundoplication, the gastroepiploic arcade may be disrupted, either purposefully or inadvertently. The presence of an intact gastroepiploic artery can be assessed preoperatively by computed tomography (CT) or conventional angiography. If the artery appears to have been compromised, the surgeon should be prepared for the use of an alternative conduit. If there is a question of whether or not the artery is intact intraoperatively, palpation and/or Doppler ultrasound can be used (open esophagectomy) or the infusion of indocyanine green with near-infrared fluorescence imaging can visualize the blood vessel (robotic or laparoscopic esophagectomy).[5]

Patients who have undergone prior weight-loss operations often pose a challenge during the surgical management of esophageal cancer, but certain situations can still afford the use of the remnant stomach for future surgical use. Review of the literature reveals that these are rare cases, but case reports have shown that these cases can still be performed using minimally invasive approaches.[6–8] Knowledge of the specific bypass procedure performed is necessary because it determines conduit and reconstruction options.[9,10]

Laparoscopic sleeve gastrectomy continues to gain popularity as a surgical intervention for weight loss with the bariatric surgical community. The American Society for Metabolic and Bariatric Surgery reports that in 2016, 125,318 laparoscopic sleeve gastrectomies were performed, accounting for 58% of all bariatric procedures performed in that year.[11] With an increase in all bariatric procedures being performed, the report also noted a 10% increase in bariatric procedures between 2011 to 2016, current trends estimate that sleeve gastrectomy will continue to be a commonly performed procedure. Notably, sleeve gastrectomy will render the stomach unusable as a future conduit for esophagectomy as the gastroepiploic artery is sacrificed. The resulting sleeve gastrectomy relies on its vascular supply from left and right gastric arteries along the lesser curvature of the remaining gastric tube, along with perforating posterior collateral branches.

In patients who have undergone Roux-en-Y gastric bypass, the remnant stomach can safely be used after lysis and release of the Roux limb. The gastric pouch is then resected with the specimen. The restoration of gastrointestinal continuity in these cases may require additional anastomoses, which would further increase the complexity and potential operative complications. Other weight-loss surgical procedures that may be encountered include band gastroplasty and other bypass procedures (duodenal switch and jejunal-ileal bypass).

Historically, the surgical management of ulcer disease included antrectomy and gastrojejunostomy, sacrificing the right gastroepiploic artery. Although current trends in upper gastrointestinal bleeding and ulcer management have reduced the need for surgery, instead now favoring endoscopic and interventional radiologic treatment, there can still be issues for future surgical inventions. Interventional management, such as embolization of the gastroduodenal artery,[12] can similarly render the stomach unusable as an option for esophageal reconstruction, because the right gastroepiploic artery arises from the gastroduodenal artery. In this group of patients, alternative conduits need to be considered.

Like patients with prior gastric surgery, intrinsic diseases of the stomach can preclude its use as a conduit. Patients with diabetic gastroparesis have poor gastric emptying at baseline and should be considered for alternative options. Use of this stomach as a conduit can have prolonged and profound diminished conduit emptying. Similarly, patients with premalignant polyps of the stomach should have an alternative conduit selected.

ALTERNATIVE CONDUITS

Familiarity with alternative conduit options is key for surgeons managing esophageal cancer. Many institutions address these patients as a collaboration between surgeons from multiple specialties that include thoracic surgeons, complex general surgical oncologists, colorectal surgeons, and/or plastic surgeons. The choice of conduit depends on the length of the gap to be spanned, the availability of conduit, and the surgeon's familiarity and comfort with the procedure (**Table 1**).

Small intestine, namely jejunum, is used commonly in esophageal reconstruction. Jejunum has been described and favored for many reasons. It has intrinsic peristalsis, possesses a luminal size comparable with that of the esophagus, is abundant and mobile, does not require significant formal preparation, has a reliable blood supply, and is

Table 1
Advantages and disadvantages of potential esophageal conduits

	Advantages	Disadvantages
Gastric conduit	• Commonly performed • Reliable blood supply • Excellent length • Single anastomosis • Easily prepared • Safe with minimally invasive methods	• Reduced reservoir • Regurgitation/reflux
Jejunal conduit	• Intrinsic peristalsis • Comparable luminal size • Abundant • Mobile • Generally free of intrinsic pathology • Does not require significant formal preparation • Can be used in several methods of reconstruction	• More complexity • Limitations in length • Need for multiple anastomoses • May require microvascular revascularization
Colonic conduit	• Adequate length • Able to function as a reservoir • Resistance to gastric acid • Reduced reflux	• More complexity • Variable blood supply • Need for multiple anastomoses • Long-term redundancy • Risk of intrinsic pathology • Requires preoperative preparation

generally free from native diseases. However, a history of inflammatory bowel disease with small bowel involvement, small bowel diverticular disease, or angiodysplasia should lead to consideration of alternative conduits. Though not routine, preoperative CT angiography has been described. The jejunum can be used with several methods for reconstruction of a conduit: as a segmental reconstruction bridging a short gap between esophagus and stomach, as a primary conduit into the midthoracic esophagus, as a pedicled jejunal interposition or free flap, or as a supercharged pedicled interposition, which can reach up to the cervical esophagus. Supercharged pedicled jejunal interposition involves anastomosis to the internal mammary artery and vein, often in conjunction with microvascular surgical specialists.[13] Consideration can be given to supercharging the distal portion of the conduit if concerns about the arterial supply are present.

Similarly, colonic conduits have also been used since the early days of esophageal reconstruction.[14] Advocates of colonic interposition cite the substantial length and resistance to gastric acid injury as advantages. Detractors often specify intrinsic diseases, need for additional anastomoses for reconstruction, and lengthening over time, which may result in redundancy, as drawbacks. Either the left or right colon can be used. The blood supply for the left colon, originating from the inferior mesentery artery, is more constant in comparison with the variable supply of the right colon, originating from the superior mesenteric artery. Interposition is oriented to facilitate an isoperistaltic intestinal anastomosis. Although rare, there have been cases reported with development of polyps or cancers in the interposed colonic segment,[15,16] which raise awareness that while no guidelines exist for surveillance of the transposed bowel, endoscopic screening strategies can be considered for these patients who undergo a change in environmental exposure to the interposed segment, along with the continued, native risk of developing disorder.

In addition to the more constant arterial supply of the left colon, it is smaller in diameter and less prone to dilatation when compared with the cecum and right colon. Proponents of the right colonic conduit cite its sufficient length and robust blood supply even in the face of anatomic variability. As such, the use of the right colon as a conduit remains an equally popular choice by many surgeons. It should be noted that in either case, right or left colon, the transverse colon is additionally harvested to provide further length.[14,17]

As opposed to a gastric or jejunal conduit, use of a colonic conduit requires preplanning. A history of ischemic insult or inflammatory bowel disease requires further investigation. In addition, patients with risk of malignancy, diverticular disease, and even polyposis are ruled out from the use of colonic interposition. Preoperative colonoscopy is routine. Other modalities, such as imaging or angiography, can be included to evaluate the patency of arterial vascular arcades. Preoperative bowel preparation is used in cases where colonic interposition is planned, and should be instituted for cases in which colonic conduits are being considered as an intraoperative alternative.

The segment of colon harvested is based on the length of the reconstruction required as well as adequate blood supply. As already mentioned, the right colon has a more variable blood supply in comparison with the left. Using the ascending and transverse colon as a graft uses the blood supply either on the ileocolic or the right colic artery. Some surgeons who favor using the right colon describe ligating right/middle colic arteries, thereby relying exclusively on the ileocolic artery. The transverse and left colon depends commonly on the left colic artery, and occasionally on the middle colic artery branches, for its supply. Intraoperatively, regardless of chosen segment, the entire colon is mobilized and the vascular supply examined.

Transillumination of the mesentery is used to locate vessels, with some advocating for a prolonged clamp trial to ensure adequate vascular supply. Division of vessels and mesentery occurs as centrally as possible.

Conduits for esophageal reconstruction can be brought via multiple positions, including tunneling from posterior mediastinal, retrosternal, or subcutaneous positions. The subcutaneous route is the longest, with the sharpest angles exiting the cervical area and re-entering the abdomen, resulting in a high rate of graft ischemia and necrosis. Therefore, it is generally reserved for cases when there are no other suitable options.[17] The posterior mediastinum is the shortest route, minimizing the length of conduit needed and the risk of ischemic complications. It is generally preferred for immediate reconstruction. In cases when the posterior mediastinum is a reoperative field, significant scarring may preclude safe access to this space. The retrosternal space has been advocated when the posterior mediastinum is not readily accessible, such as in cases of delayed esophageal reconstruction or in palliative cases. Creating the retrosternal tunnel does not require a thoracic incision, thereby minimizing pulmonary complications. Creation of the proximal anastomosis in the cervical region can lead to compression and ischemia of the conduit, and it is generally advisable to widen the thoracic inlet by resecting the left hemimanubrium, clavicular head, and portion of the first rib. Additionally this allows access to the left internal mammary vessels in cases where microvascular anastomoses are required.

INTRAOPERATIVE ISSUES AND POSTOPERATIVE LEAKS

Another concern for esophageal surgeons is intraoperative difficulty or concerns with the conduit. Intraoperative evaluation with fluorescence angiography or Doppler evaluation of the blood supply for the graft has been described to identify ischemia. For example, laparoscopic or robotic evaluation with indocyanine green and near-infrared optimal imaging has been a useful adjunct.[18,19] To this end, 5 to 10 mg of indocyanine green is given intravenously. The conduit can then be assessed for perfusion in a qualitative fashion, as the indocyanine green is distributed in the tissue. This information can be used during creation of the conduit and locating where the anastomosis will be performed on the gastric wall. If the conduit does not have adequate length, there are further options. As noted earlier, segmental jejunal interposition can be used to overcome difficulty in length. In the situation where the conduit is completely ischemic, consideration can be given to leaving the patient in discontinuity for 24 to 72 hours and then returning to the operating room to re-evaluate, thus allowing for demarcation of ischemic regions. Similarly, some surgeons would advocate for diversion with a cervical esophagostomy and enteric feeding access, and return at a later date to allow the patient time to recover and receive additional necessary oncologic treatments.

There are many postoperative complications that can arise in patients who have undergone esophagectomy, but anastomotic leak remains one of the most dreaded. Intrathoracic anastomoses were thought historically to have lower leak rates, but higher morbidity when compared with cervical anastomoses, which were thought to have a higher rate of postoperative leak but less morbidity.[20,21] Using the stomach as the conduit has the lowest reported incidence of conduit ischemia, followed by jejunum and the colon. In addition, the technique of anastomosis plays a role in postoperative anastomotic leak. A review of anastomotic techniques reveals that hand-sewn anastomoses have a higher incidence of leak than multiple stapled techniques.[22] Although a variety of techniques exist and there is an overall lack of consensus regarding the optimal method, an important technical consideration is ensuring mucosal inclusion throughout the anastomosis.

Diagnosing anastomotic leaks after esophagectomy remains an area of difficulty, with variable methods of diagnoses affecting reporting and management. Similarly, owing to the difference in definitions, grading systems, and treatment algorithms used throughout the literature, comparison between studies is difficult. There are several classifications available to grade anastomotic leaks. A common system was developed by Lerut and colleagues.[23] Methods of diagnosis involve surgeon and institution preference, ranging from clinical to radiographic (fluoroscopic, cross-sectional imaging), to endoscopic evaluations.

Managing conduit leaks after esophagectomy requires stratification of treatment options based on the severity of leak along with the patient's clinical condition, the location of anastomosis, the type of conduit used, and the method of anastomosis. Clinically stable patients with occult anastomotic leaks discovered only by imaging can be managed by delaying oral intake. Leaks with signs of infection should be managed with antibiotic therapy, adequate drainage of the cavity, and reduction of gastric acid secretion with proton-pump inhibitors and somatostatin treatment.[24] Stenting has also been found to be an effective method to manage anastomotic leaks, providing occlusion of the leak. Endoscopic intervention allows the opportunity for earlier oral intake while avoiding repeat operations.[25] In cervical anastomoses, drainage can be achieved by opening the incision at bedside, whereas intrathoracic anastomoses may require radiologically guided or potentially surgical drainage. In all cases of anastomotic leaks, focus should additionally remain on maintaining adequate nutritional support via enteral or parenteral routes.

The rare and feared complication of conduit necrosis (classified as Lerut grade IV) after esophagectomy requires a multifactorial approach. Surgical management includes source control by resecting the nonviable segment of the conduit, proximal esophageal diversion while preserving esophageal length when possible, and returning any remaining viable conduit to the abdomen. Further management includes antimicrobial coverage and optimization of nutritional status. Reconstruction in the same setting is not recommended, with most surgeons preferring to operate in a delayed fashion after recovery and often via alternative routes.[26,27]

With focused attention to surgical techniques and diagnosing and managing complications, there has been an overall decline in mortality from anastomotic leaks.[28] Prevention of anastomotic complications involves a multidisciplinary approach of managing patient factors, technical considerations, and postoperative attention.

Surgery will remain a part of the multimodality treatment of esophageal cancer. Surgeons who are treating these patients will be approached with complex cases, requiring knowledge of management of the difficult esophageal conduit, alternative conduit options, and intraoperative issues. Continued advancements in postoperative management will also enhance patient outcomes.

REFERENCES

1. Siegel RL, Miller KD, Jemal A. Cancer statistics, 2018. CA Cancer J Clin 2018; 68(1):7–30.

2. Wright GP, Foster SM, Chung MH. Esophagectomy in patients with prior percutaneous gastrostomy tube placement. Am J Surg 2014;207(3):361–5.

3. Shen KR, Harrison-Phipps KM, Cassivi SD, et al. Esophagectomy after anti-reflux surgery. J Thorac Cardiovasc Surg 2010;139(4):969–75.

4. Chang AC, Lee JS, Sawicki KT, et al. Outcomes after esophagectomy in patients with prior antireflux or hiatal hernia surgery. Ann Thorac Surg 2010;89(4): 1015–23.

5. Yukaya T, Saeki H, Kasagi Y, et al. Indocyanine green fluorescence angiography for quantitative evaluation of gastric tube perfusion in patients undergoing esophagectomy. J Am Coll Surg 2015;221:e37–42.

6. Rossidis G, Browning R, Hochwald SN, et al. Minimally invasive esophagectomy is safe in patients with previous gastric bypass. Surg Obes Relat Dis 2014;10(1): 95–100.

7. Kuruba R, Jawad M, Karl RC, et al. Technique of resection of esophageal adenocarcinoma after Roux-en-Y gastric bypass and literature review of esophagogastric tumors after bariatric procedures. Surg Obes Relat Dis 2009;5(5):576–81.

8. Allen JW, Leeman MF, Richardson JD. Esophageal carcinoma following bariatric procedures. JSLS 2004;8(4):372–5.

9. Nguyen NT, Tran C, Gelfand DV, et al. Laparoscopic and thoracoscopic Ivor Lewis esophagectomy after Roux-en-Y gastric bypass. Ann Thorac Surg 2006; 82(5):1910–3.

10. Marino KA, Weksler B. Esophagectomy after weight-reduction surgery. Thorac Surg Clin 2018;28(1):53–8.

11. English WJ, DeMaria EJ, Brethauer SA, et al. American Society for Metabolic and Bariatric Surgery estimation of metabolic and bariatric procedures performed in the United States in 2016. Surg Obes Relat Dis 2018;14:259.

12. Shin JH. Recent update of embolization of upper gastrointestinal tract bleeding. Korean J Radiol 2012;13(Suppl 1):S31–9.

13. Blackmon SH, Correa AM, Skoracki R, et al. Supercharged pedicled jejunal interposition for esophageal replacement: a 10-year experience. Ann Thorac Surg 2012;94(4):1104–11.

14. Bakshi A, Sugarbaker DJ, Burt BM. Alternative conduits for esophageal replacement. Ann Cardiothorac Surg 2017;6(2):137–43.

15. Aryal MR, Mainali NR, Jalota L, et al. Advanced adenocarcinoma in a colonic interposition segment. BMJ Case Rep 2013;2013. bcr2013009749.

16. Altomare JF, Komar MJ. A tubular adenoma arising in a colonic interposition. J Clin Gastroenterol 2006;2013:765–6.

17. Boukerrouche A. Colon reconstruction and esophageal reconstructive surgery. Med Clin Rev 2016;2:27. https://doi.org/10.21767/2471-299X.1000036.

18. Sarkaria IS, Bains MS, Finley DJ, et al. Intraoperative near-infrared fluorescence imaging as an adjunct to robotic assisted minimally invasive esophagectomy. Innovations (Phila) 2014;9(5):391–3.

19. Zehtner J, DeMeester SR, Alicuben ET, et al. Intraoperative assessment of perfusion of the gastric graft and correlation with anastomotic leaks after esophagectomy. Ann Surg 2015;262(1):74–8.

20. Kassis ES, Kosinki AS, Ross P, et al. Predictors of anastomotic leak after esophagectomy: an analysis of the society of thoracic surgeons general thoracic database. Ann Thorac Surg 2013;96:1919–26.

21. Giuli R, Gignoux M. Treatment of carcinoma of the esophagus: retrospective study of 2,400 patients. Ann Surg 1980;192:44–52.

22. Price TN, Nichols FC, Harmsen WS, et al. A comprehensive review of anastomotic techniques in 432 esophagectomies. Ann Thorac Surg 2013;95:1154–61.

23. Lerut T, Coosemans W, Decker G, et al. Anastomotic complications after esophagectomy. Dig Surg 2002;19(2):92–8.

24. Meyerson SL, Mehta CK. Managing complications II: conduit failure and conduit airway fistulas. J Thorac Dis 2014;6(Supple 3):S364–71.
25. Freeman RK, Vyverberg A, Ascioti AJ. Esophageal stent placement for the treatment of acute intrathoracic anastomotic leak after esophagectomy. Ann Thorac Surg 2011;9(2):204–8.
26. Wormuth JK, Heitmiller RF. Esophageal conduit necrosis. Thorac Surg Clin 2006; 16:11–22.
27. Dickinson KJ, Blackmon SH. Management of conduit necrosis following esophagectomy. Thorac Surg Clin 2015;25:461–70.
28. Martin LW, Swisher SG, Hofstetter W, et al. Intrathoracic leaks following esophagectomy are no longer associated with increased mortality. Ann Surg 2005;242: 392–402.

Combined Modality Therapy for Management of Esophageal Cancer

Current Approach Based on Experiences from East and West

Omeed Moaven, MD[a], Thomas N. Wang, MD, PhD[b],*

KEYWORDS

- Esophageal adenocarcinoma • Esophageal squamous cell carcinoma
- Multimodality therapy • Definitive chemoradiation • Lymphadenectomy

KEY POINTS

- Esophageal cancer is more prevalent in Eastern countries, predominantly in the form of esophageal squamous cell carcinoma. In contrast, the pattern is more mixed in Western countries, with esophageal adenocarcinoma being the more frequent subtype.
- Advancements in systemic treatment have shifted the therapeutic paradigm in esophageal cancer toward multimodality treatment in recent decades.
- Treatment strategy is more standardized in Western countries.
- Various surgical approaches of esophagectomy have similar overall outcomes with no clear benefit of one technique over the others.
- For patients who are not operative candidates or who wish to avoid surgery, definitive chemoradiation has been shown to be a promising modality in a subgroup of patients. Salvage surgery has been shown to be a feasible option in those who fail or recur with nonsurgical management.

INTRODUCTION

The first successful esophagectomy for cancer was performed a century ago in Germany, and the patient survived 12 years.[1] Since then, knowledge of cancer biology and advancements in nonsurgical modalities, including chemotherapy and radiation, have led to the evolution of therapeutic strategies through the multimodality approach

Disclosures: The authors have no relevant disclosures.
[a] Division of Surgical Oncology, Department of Surgery, Wake Forest University, Medical Center Boulevard, Winston-Salem, NC 27157, USA; [b] Division of Surgical Oncology, Department of Surgery, University of Alabama at Birmingham, BDB 609, 1808 7th Avenue South, Birmingham, AL 35294-3411, USA
* Corresponding author.
E-mail address: thomaswang@uabmc.edu

for the treatment of esophageal cancer. Esophageal cancer has discrete regional characteristics as a result of diverse environmental exposures and distinct genetic alterations. The evolutionary divergence in the geographic distribution of genetic variations has led to various differences in epidemiology, molecular signature, and clinical behavior of esophageal cancer, subsequently resulting in differences in management of this disease. Thus, the basis of discrete approaches in the management of esophageal cancer between Eastern versus Western countries is caused by the differences in their tumor biology and pathologic behavior. This article discusses the distinct epidemiologic and molecular characteristics of esophageal cancer across the world and the Eastern and Western perspectives in multimodality therapy for esophageal cancer.

EPIDEMIOLOGY

Esophageal cancer is the eighth most common malignancy worldwide, predominantly distributed in developing countries, and has the sixth highest incidence in cancer mortality. Esophageal cancer has a male predilection with a ratio of 2:1.[2] Although the incidence of esophageal cancer has been declining in Eastern countries, the trend in Western countries is more varied. The incidence of esophageal cancer has increased in English and Danish men; remained stable in men from the United States, Canada, and Australia; and decreased in French men. The overall incidence has remained stable among women in Western countries.[2]

Esophageal cancer is divided into 2 major histologic subtypes: adenocarcinoma (AC) and squamous cell carcinoma (SCC). Each histologic subtype has distinct clinicopathologic and demographic characteristics. SCC is the more commonly seen histologic subtype worldwide, predominantly found in Eastern countries, although its overall incidence is declining. SCC has a greater predilection for the proximal esophagus and is generally associated with tobacco smoking, alcohol consumption, and low socioeconomic status.[3] In contrast, there has been a significant increase in the prevalence of AC, which is more frequently seen in Western countries. The major risk factors for the development of AC include gastroesophageal reflux disease and the presence of Barrett esophagus.[4,5]

Squamous Cell Carcinoma

A plethora of causal factors contribute to the carcinogenesis of SCC. These factors are strongly population dependent, and there is a distinct variation between Eastern and Western populations. In a multicenter population-based study evaluating individuals with SCC in the United States, factors with high population-attributable risks (PARs) for SCC included heavy alcohol use, tobacco smoking, and the inadequate consumption of fruits and vegetables.[6] In contrast, a prospective study from China showed that smoking has only a modest impact on the development of SCC, and drinking alcohol was not associated with an increased risk.[7] Low socioeconomic status is a strong risk factor consistently shown to increase the risk of SCC in both developing and developed countries worldwide.[8] Smoking seems to be a stronger risk factors in Western countries.[8] The reported relative risk is consistently higher in multiple Western patient population studies (3-fold to 5-fold in smokers).[9–11] In contrast, cohorts studies from Eastern countries with high esophageal cancer incidence, including China and Iran, report a lesser impact from tobacco use (relative risk <2).[7,12] Similarly, alcohol consumption is also a stronger risk factor in Western countries. Engel and colleagues[6] reported a PAR fraction of 72.4% (95% confidence interval], 53.3% to 85.8%) for alcohol consumption, whereas PAR fraction for alcohol consumption was only 10.9% in a cohort published from China.[13] Consumption of fresh fruit and vegetables has been shown to exert a protective role against SCC in both Eastern and Western studies. Drinking hot beverages and food has been shown to be a risk factor in studies from Asia (China and Iran) and South America (Brazil, Argentina, Uruguay, and Paraguay).[14–17] Other risk factors, such as poor oral hygiene, opium use, and polycyclic aromatic hydrocarbon exposure, have also been shown to be associated with an increased risk of SCC in various studies, but further studies are required to validate the causal relationship between these factors and SCC carcinogenesis.[18]

Adenocarcinoma

Most epidemiologic studies on esophageal AC are cohort studies from Western countries. Gastroesophageal reflux disease and Barrett esophagus are well-established risk factors for the development of AC in Western countries, and their association to AC is stronger in young patients.[19,20] In a meta-analysis of 51 previous studies, Shiota and colleagues[21] reported that Barrett esophagus is common in Eastern countries, and its risk factor for the development of AC is similar to that of Western countries. Obesity and abdominal adiposity have also been shown to play a role in AC development with a significant linear dose-response association.[22,23] However, neither medications to decrease acid reflux nor weight loss surgeries have been shown to decrease the risk of AC development.[4] Smoking has also been shown to increase the risk of AC development, with a lower relative risk in the development of AC (2-fold to 3-fold) compared with SCC in Western countries.[24] Smoking cessation for greater than 10 years in long-term smokers can reduce the risk of AC development by 30% to 40% compared with individuals who continue to smoke.[25] In contrast, alcohol consumption has not been shown to increase the risk of AC.[26]

EASTERN PERSPECTIVE ON COMBINED MODALITY THERAPY
Surgical Multimodality Approach: Neoadjuvant Therapy

Radiotherapy
Radiotherapy as a single-modality neoadjuvant approach has not been shown to be an effective treatment strategy. Several randomized trials failed to prove a survival benefit for patients who received radiation therapy before surgery compared with surgery alone.[27,28]

Chemotherapy
Preoperative chemotherapy with cisplatin/5-fluorouracil (5-FU) is accepted as the standard of care in Japan. Several randomized neoadjuvant chemotherapy trials previously showed inconclusive evidence for this treatment strategy for esophageal cancer.[29–31] The Japan Clinical Oncology Group (JCOG) 9907 trial showed a survival benefit with neoadjuvant chemotherapy (cisplatin, 5-FU).[32] In this trial, 330 patients with SCC with stage II and III (excluding T4) were randomized to either preoperative or postoperative chemotherapy with 2 cycles of cisplatin and 5-FU. Progression-free survival and overall survival were significantly better in the neoadjuvant group. However, a meta-analysis pooling data from 6 randomized trials, including JCOG 9907, performed by Zheng and colleagues[33] failed to show any survival benefit for neoadjuvant chemotherapy. Presently, a phase III trial is ongoing to investigate the survival benefit of neoadjuvant cisplatin plus paclitaxel versus surgery alone in China (ClinicalTrials.gov identifier: NCT02395705).

Chemoradiotherapy
Neoadjuvant chemoradiation has not been widely adopted as the preferred combined therapeutic modality for the treatment of SCC. **Table 1** represents available

Table 1
Randomized trials comparing preoperative chemoradiation versus surgery alone for esophageal squamous cell carcinoma in Eastern countries

Authors, Year	Country	Sample Size	pCR	Survival Rate	P Value
Apinop et al,[114] 1994	Thailand	CRS 35 vs SA 34	20%	24% vs 10% (5 y)	NS
An et al,[34] 2003	China	CRS 48 vs SA 49	56.5%	56.7% (CRS, 5 y)	.035
Lee et al,[36] 2004	Korea	CRS 51 vs SA 50	43%	55% vs 57% (2 y)	NS
Natsugoe et al,[37] 2006	Japan	CRS 22 vs SA 23	15%	57% vs 41% (5 y)	NS
Cao et al,[35] 2009	China	CRS 118 vs SA 118	22.3%	73% vs 53% (3 y)	<.01
Yang et al,[38] 2018	China	CRS 224 vs SA 227	43.2%	69% vs 59% (3 y)	.025

Abbreviations: CRS, chemoradiation followed by surgery; NS, not significant; pCR, pathologic complete response; SA, surgery alone.

randomized trials that have compared preoperative chemoradiation versus surgery alone. The older trials have been criticized for the inadequacy of the systemic treatments used.[34–37] Yang and colleagues[38] recently reported the results of a phase III randomized clinical trial (NEOCRTEC5010) comparing preoperative chemoradiation followed by surgery versus surgery alone. They randomized 451 patients with locally advanced SCC (T1-4N1M0/T4N0M0) into a preoperative chemoradiation group and a surgery-alone group. The preoperative chemoradiation group received 2 cycles of vinorelbine and cisplatin and a total of 40.0 Gy of radiation in 20 fractions. Preoperative chemoradiation resulted in 43.2% pathologic complete response and a superior R0 resection rate (98.4% vs 91.2%). Preoperative chemoradiation significantly improved median survival (100.1 months vs 66.5 months), disease-free survival (100.1 months vs 41.7 months), and 3-year overall survival (69.1% vs 58.9%). In a multivariate analysis, preoperative chemoradiation was an independent factor in improved overall survival. In addition, a meta-analysis of 43 published randomized clinical trials by Doosti-Irani and colleagues[39] showed that neoadjuvant chemoradiation with carboplatin and paclitaxel followed by surgery provided the most improved survival benefit among the various neoadjuvant and adjuvant multimodality treatment strategies in SCC.

To date, Japanese surgeons have been reluctant to accept the results of the multiple prospective studies and meta-analyses showing the superiority of preoperative chemoradiation to preoperative chemotherapy, citing the results of JCOG 9907 and the belief that their superior outcomes may be caused by the differences in their patient population tumor biology and their surgical techniques. In order to study the multimodality therapy with the best efficacy for their patient population, Japanese investigators have initiated a 3-armed phase III randomized trial (JCOG1109) comparing the standard preoperative chemotherapy (cisplatin, 5-FU) with an enhanced preoperative chemotherapy (docetaxel, cisplatin, 5-FU) and a preoperative chemoradiation therapy regimen (cisplatin, 5-FU plus radiation).[40]

Surgical Multimodality Approach: Adjuvant Therapy

Radiotherapy

Postoperative radiotherapy (without chemotherapy) was not shown to provide a survival benefit in SCC compared with surgery alone in 4 published trials, 2 of which were completed in Western countries.[41–44] In a randomized clinical trial performed by Fok and colleagues[41] comparing patients treated with postoperative radiation therapy versus surgery alone, overall survival for patients treated with adjuvant radiation therapy (49.5 Gy) was significantly worse. The largest randomized clinical trial was conducted by Xiao and colleagues,[42] who randomized 495 patients to adjuvant radiation therapy versus surgery alone. The investigators found no survival difference between the two groups.

Chemotherapy

Ando and colleagues[45] conducted JCOG 9204, in which 242 patients with SCC were randomized into 2 groups: surgery followed by 2 cycles of cisplatin plus 5-FU versus surgery alone. Although disease-free survival was improved in the group that received adjuvant treatment, the overall survival between the two groups was not different. This study was followed by the JCOG 9907 trial, which showed the superiority of preoperative over postoperative chemotherapy as previously mentioned.[32] The results of JCOG 9907 will remain the basis for the standard of care in Japan unless the results of JCOG 1109 determine a better preoperative treatment strategy.[46]

Chemoradiation

No randomized trial has compared the addition of chemoradiation postoperatively with esophagectomy alone.

Nonsurgical Approach: Definitive Chemoradiation

Definitive chemoradiation is the standard treatment of patients with unresectable esophageal malignancies, patients who are poor surgical candidates, and patients who refuse surgical treatment. Most studies evaluating the efficacy of definitive chemoradiation for resectable disease have been nonrandomized studies.[47–55] Teoh and colleagues[56] conducted the only randomized clinical trial in Eastern countries. The investigators randomized 81 patients with resectable midesophageal or distal esophageal SCC into 2 groups: esophagectomy or definitive chemoradiation therapy. There was no significant difference between the two groups with respect to disease-free survival or overall survival. Although not significant, the investigators observed a trend favoring definitive chemoradiation in the 5-year overall survival for patients with node-positive disease ($P = .061$). Ma and colleagues[57] performed a meta-analysis of the current literature and showed a similar result between esophagectomy and definitive chemoradiation. However, most of the included studies were nonrandomized and retrospective studies with the inherent selection biases.

Kato and colleagues[58] reported the efficacy of chemoradiation for stage II and III SCC as a definitive therapeutic modality with a complete response of 62.2%, a median survival of 29 months, and a 3-year and 5-year survival rate of 44.7% and 36.7% respectively (JCOG 9906). Although these results are inferior to the standard surgical treatment, it provides a reasonable nonsurgical option for those who wish to avoid or cannot tolerate esophagectomy. In another phase II study (JCOG 9708), Kato and colleagues[59] evaluated the efficacy of definitive chemoradiation in stage I SCC. Seventy-two patients with node-negative, T1 tumors were treated with combined modality chemotherapy (cisplatin, 5-FU) and 30-Gy radiotherapy. A complete response required meeting all of the following criteria: (1) no evidence of tumor except flat erosion, flat fur, or a scar; (2) a negative biopsy; (3) no new lesions; and (4) confirmation of (1) to (3) with at least a 4-week interval. Sixty-three patients had a complete response (87.5%). Among the patients with residual disease after treatment, 6 underwent successful esophagectomy. Although lacking sufficient high-level evidence, the present studies suggest that definitive chemoradiation may be equivalent to surgery in the treatment of patients with early SCC. An ongoing phase III trial (JCOG 0502) in Japan is designed to determine once and for all whether esophagectomy is necessary for patients with SCC who are complete responders after definitive chemoradiation.

Salvage Surgery

For patients with residual disease or recurrent disease after chemoradiation therapy, salvage surgery is the recommended treatment option in the East.[60] However, surgeons are often reluctant to pursue this approach because of the significantly higher morbidity and mortality associated with salvage surgery.[61] Nevertheless, it can provide long-term survival benefits in highly selected patients. No randomized trial has compared salvage surgery with second-line chemotherapy. Kumagai and colleagues[62] reported a meta-analysis of 4 retrospective studies comparing survival and treatment-related mortality in patients submitted to salvage esophagectomy or second-line chemotherapy for recurrent or persistent SCC after definitive chemoradiation. There was a long-term survival benefit for patients undergoing esophagectomy, with a pooled hazard ratio (HR) for death of 0.42 for salvage surgery compared with second-line chemoradiotherapy ($P = .017$). However, salvage esophagectomy was associated with a treatment-related mortality of 10.3% in the 36 patients who underwent resection. Thus, salvage esophagectomy may provide a significant gain in long-term survival compared with second-line chemoradiotherapy but at the cost of a high treatment-related mortality. JCOG 0909 is an ongoing nonrandomized study that is designed to investigate the efficacy of definitive chemoradiation with or without salvage surgery for patients with stage II and III disease.

WESTERN PERSPECTIVE ON COMBINED-MODALITY THERAPY
Surgical Multimodality Approach: Neoadjuvant Therapy

Radiotherapy

Arnott and colleagues[63] reported the only randomized clinical trial comparing radiation therapy followed by surgery with surgery alone for AC. The investigators showed that the addition of preoperative radiation provided no added benefit to resection. Likewise, other Western clinical trials showed similar findings when comparing neoadjuvant radiation therapy versus surgery alone for the treatment of SCC.[28,64] In a meta-analysis, pooling data from 5 randomized trials comprising 1147 patients with SCC, Arnott and colleagues[65] also failed to show a significant survival benefit for patients treated with neoadjuvant radiation for potentially resectable disease. In addition, the results of Radiation Therapy Oncology Group 85-01 (RTOG 85-01) trial provides additional evidence that chemoradiation is superior to radiation alone in the treatment of esophageal cancer, although both arms of this trial did not include surgery.[66]

Chemotherapy

Several Western randomized trials have compared preoperative chemotherapy versus surgery alone in the treatment of both SCC and AC. Roth and colleagues[67] published the first Western trial, showing that preoperative chemotherapy did not provide a survival benefit compared with surgery alone. However, the trial did show that the subset of complete responders to systemic therapy did show a survival advantage. Two other trials from Germany and Italy also failed to show a survival benefit for patients with SCC treated with preoperative chemotherapy.[68,69] In contrast, a Medical Research Council (MRC) phase III trial from the United Kingdom showed that neoadjuvant chemotherapy (2 cycles of cisplatin, 5-FU) improved the R0 resection rate and the overall survival rate in patients with both SCC and AC.[70] Long-term results of this trial further confirmed the continued benefit of preoperative chemotherapy.[71] Four meta-analyses have pooled the results of published trials. Two of them did not show any survival benefit for neoadjuvant chemotherapy.[72,73] Another systemic review, the

Cochrane Review, compared survivals at various time points from 1 to 5 years. Although the survival was not different in the first 4 years, 5-year survival was better when preoperative chemotherapy was administered.[74] The review was updated in 2015 and showed that preoperative chemotherapy improved the overall survival rate and the R0 resection rate. However, the evidence for a survival advantage in patients treated with preoperative chemotherapy is considered of moderate quality.[75]

Kelson and colleagues[76] reported the results of RTOG 8911 (North American Intergroup 0113) comparing preoperative chemotherapy (3 cycles of cisplatin, 5-FU) or adjuvant chemotherapy (2 cycles, cisplatin, 5-FU) with esophagectomy alone for SCC and AC. The investigators found no survival benefit in the patients treated with systemic therapy. However, the compliance was suboptimal, with only 68% of the neoadjuvant group and 38% of the adjuvant group completing the intended chemotherapy regimen. The landmark trial addressing preoperative and postoperative chemotherapy is the MRC Adjuvant Gastric Infusion Chemotherapy (MAGIC) trial, in which systemic therapy (cisplatin, 5-FU, epirubicin) was administered preoperatively and postoperatively (3 cycles each). Enrolled patients included predominantly patients with gastric cancer; however, there was a subgroup of patients with esophagogastric junction and esophageal cancer. The trial showed improved overall and progression-free survival in the patients who received chemotherapy.[77] The results of the MAGIC trial have become the basis for the recommended treatment of resectable gastric cancer in most Western centers but has not been adopted for the treatment of resectable esophageal cancer.

Chemoradiation

Preoperative chemoradiation is presently the standard of practice in Western countries for resectable SCC or AC with or without regional lymph node metastasis. Several trials have investigated the role of preoperative chemoradiation compared with surgery alone (**Table 2**). These studies have been criticized for various weaknesses, including the choice of chemotherapy regimens, the dose of radiation, poor accrual, underpowered studies, and poor surgical outcomes. The landmark trial that has

Table 2
Randomized trials comparing preoperative chemoradiation versus surgery alone for esophageal adenocarcinoma and esophageal squamous cell carcinoma in Western countries

Authors, Year	Country	Sample Size	Histology	Survival Rate	P Value
Nygaard et al,[115] 1992	Scandinavian MC	CRS 53 vs SA 50	ESCC	17% vs 9% (3 y)	NS
Le Prise et al,[116] 1994	France	CRS 41 vs SA 45	ESCC	19% vs 14% (3 y)	NS
Walsh et al,[117] 1996	Ireland	CRS 58 vs SA 55	EA	32% vs 6% (3 y)	.010
Bosset et al,[118] 1997	France	CRS 143 vs SA 139	ESCC	33% vs 32% (5 y)	NS
Urba et al,[119] 2001	USA	CRS 50 vs SA 50	ESCC + EA	20% vs 10% (5 y)	NS
Tepper et al,[120] 2008 (CALGB 9781)	USA	CRS 30 vs SA 26	ESCC + EA	39% vs 16% (5 y)	.002
Van Hagen et al,[78] 2012 (CROSS)	Netherlands	CRS 178 vs SA 188	ESCC + EA	47% vs 34% (5 y)	.003

Abbreviations: EA, esophageal AC; ESCC, esophageal SCC; MC, multicenter.

established neoadjuvant chemoradiation as the standard practice for the treatment of resectable esophageal cancer is the Chemoradiotherapy for Oesophageal Cancer Followed by Surgery Study (CROSS) trial.[78] van Hagen and colleagues[78] randomized 178 patients with resectable disease to neoadjuvant chemoradiation and 188 patients to surgery alone over a period of 4 years. Of the 366 patients analyzed, 75% had AC, 23% had SCC, and 2% had undifferentiated cancers. Patients in the neoadjuvant therapy arm were treated with carboplatin and paclitaxel for 5 weeks in combination with radiation (41.4 Gy in 23 fractions). The toxicity was acceptable, with leukopenia the most common hematologic side effect (6%) and anorexia the most common nonhematologic side effect (5%). R0 resection was significantly higher in the combined modality group (92% vs 69%; $P<.001$). Of those who completed chemoradiation, 29% (47 out of 161) achieved a pathologic complete response. This response was significantly higher in patients with SCC compared with esophageal AC (49% vs 23%; $P = .008$). Nodal involvement was also significantly lower in the multimodality group compared with the surgery-alone group (75% vs 31%; $P<.001$). Median overall survival was significantly higher in the multimodality group (49.4 months vs 24 months; HR, 0.66; $P = .003$). Five-year survival was also higher in the multimodality group (47% vs 34%; HR, 0.66; $P = .003$). Shapiro and colleagues,[79] in a follow-up report, extended the median follow-up from 45 months in the original report to 84 months and again illustrated the survival benefit for preoperative chemoradiation, which was again more prominent in the patients with SCC. Median survival for SCC was 81.6 months for the multimodality group versus 21.1 months for the surgery-alone group (HR, 0.48; $P = .008$). Median survival for AC was 43.2 months versus 27.1 months (HR, 0.73; $P = .038$). In another study, 208 patients from CROSS were retrospectively compared with a cohort of 173 post-CROSS patients. This cohort included patients who were older, had higher comorbidities, and had poorer performance status. There were no differences in significant adverse events and survival rates, validating the efficacy of neoadjuvant chemoradiation followed by esophagectomy in patients with esophageal cancer.[80]

Surgical Multimodality Approach: Adjuvant Therapy

Radiotherapy
As mentioned earlier, 2 Western trials have compared the addition of postoperative radiation to surgery alone. Neither showed a survival benefit for adjuvant radiotherapy. In contrast with Eastern trials, these studies did not exclude patients with celiac node involvement (M1).[43,44]

Chemotherapy
Postoperative chemotherapy has been selectively administered for patients with distal esophageal AC and gastroesophageal junction tumors as part of a perioperative regimen. These recommendations are based on the MAGIC trial[77] and the FNCLCC/FFCD trial, which was a phase III randomized trial in 28 French centers initiated by the Fédération Nationale des Centers de Lutte Contre le Cancer (FNCLCC) and the Fédération Francophone de Cancérologie Digestive (FFCD).[81] However, most patients had gastric or gastroesophageal junction tumors, and only 25 patients (11.1%) had esophageal cancers. Postoperative chemotherapy has not been proved to improve survival in Western trials.[82]

Chemoradiation
Although adjuvant chemoradiation has benefitted gastroesophageal junction AC, there has not been a study performed to evaluate the efficacy of adjuvant chemoradiation in only esophageal cancer.

Nonsurgical Approach: Definitive Chemoradiation

Multiple trials have investigated optimal combinations for nonsurgical management of esophageal cancer in Western countries. Herskovic and colleagues[66] conducted the RTOG 85-01 trial comparing chemoradiation with radiation only in the treatment of nonmetastatic SCC or AC. There was a significantly higher 2-year survival in the chemoradiation group (38% vs 10%; $P = .001$). Cooper and colleagues[83] reported the long-term outcomes of RTOG 85-01, including 73 additional patients to the chemoradiation arm in a nonrandomized fashion. Although none of the patients from the radiation arm remained alive after 5 years, the 5-year survival was 26% for the randomized and 14% for the nonrandomized patients. In an attempt to improve the long-term outcomes and decrease the extent of locoregional disease, Intergroup 0123/RTOG 94-05 added induction chemotherapy to the chemoradiation arm and increased the radiation dose (from 50.4 Gy to 64.8 Gy). However, the outcomes did not improve and the toxicity worsened.[84]

FFCD 9102, reported by Bedenne and colleagues,[85] compared esophagectomy with further chemoradiation after induction chemoradiation. All the patients before randomization received concomitant 5-FU/cisplatin and radiation, and those who responded were randomized to either esophagectomy or additional chemoradiation. There was no difference between the median survival of the two arms, suggesting that the patients who responded to induction chemoradiation did not benefit from an esophagectomy. Despite advancements in diagnostic tools, follow-up of these patients and detection of residual disease and recurrence remains a clinical challenge. Although definitive chemoradiation is a viable option for patients who show a good response to chemoradiation, better diagnostic tests are needed to accurately identify the subset of patients who have no residual disease after induction chemoradiation and do not benefit from resection. Presently, only the pathologic evaluation of a resected specimen can make the determination of a complete response.

Salvage surgery in patients who fail to respond to definitive chemoradiation was investigated in RTOG 0246, which was a phase II nonrandomized study that showed a 5-year survival of 41% for patients with SCC and AC who had incomplete response and underwent salvage surgical resection.[86] This trial proved the feasibility of definitive chemotherapy and salvage surgery; however, larger randomized trials are necessary to validate these findings.

SURGERY, THE MAINSTAY OF COMBINED MODALITY TREATMENT

To date, the cornerstone of multimodality management of esophageal cancer is esophagectomy. The principals of surgical resection include (1) creation of a conduit, (2) adequate mobilization of the esophagus, (3) margin-negative resection of the esophagus, (4) appropriate lymphadenectomy, and (5) performance of a tension-free anastomosis. Several approaches have been introduced for the surgical management of esophageal cancer, and although each approach has its own advantages and disadvantages, no trials have proved one to be superior to the others. The decision as to which approach is selected depends on the location of the tumor, the patient's comorbidities, the available conduits, and the surgeon's experience.

The transthoracic method (Ivor Lewis) is the most commonly used approach, which consists of the intra-abdominal mobilization of the conduit followed by a right thoracotomy with an intrathoracic anastomosis. The transhiatal esophagectomy starts with a laparotomy followed by a left cervical incision with blunt dissection of the esophagus. This technique does not include a thoracotomy. In addition, a 3-field esophagectomy, or McKeown approach, consists of a laparotomy, thoracotomy, and cervical incision. For both the transhiatal esophagectomy and the McKeown procedure, the anastomosis is performed through the cervical incision. The postulated advantages of the Ivor Lewis and McKeown approaches are direct visualization of the thoracic esophagus with the potential for a more extensive lymphadenectomy. The disadvantages may include the cardiopulmonary complications of a thoracotomy and the grim consequences of an intrathoracic anastomotic leak.[87] In contrast, the transhiatal esophagectomy avoids the potential complications of a thoracotomy and an intrathoracic anastomotic leak but may result in a suboptimal oncologic resection with inadequate lymph node staging. Leak rates are higher but less devastating in the transhiatal approach. However, prospective trials and multiple meta-analyses comparing these approaches have not shown a significant difference in long-term outcome.[88–92] In the most commonly referenced randomized control trial, Hulscher and colleagues[91,92] compared 114 patients who underwent a transthoracic esophagectomy with extended lymphadenectomy with 106 patients who underwent a transhiatal esophagectomy. After a median follow-up of 4.7 years, the investigators showed that the perioperative morbidity was higher in the transthoracic esophagectomy group but there was no significant difference in in-hospital mortality ($P = .45$). Although there was no significant difference in survival between the two groups, there was a trend toward a survival benefit at 5 years in the transthoracic esophagectomy group compared with the transhiatal group in both overall survival (39% vs 29%) and disease-free survival (39% vs 27%). McKeown esophagectomy applies 3 incisions with the idea of having a cervical anastomosis to decrease morbidity of a thoracic leak while maintaining the capability to extend lymph node dissection for a better oncologic outcome. The outcomes of this technique have been shown to be similar to other techniques as well.[93] Minimally invasive surgery has been incorporated into various steps of an esophagectomy in the approaches mentioned earlier. Straatman and colleagues[94] reported the results of the multicenter, randomized TIME (Traditional Invasive versus Minimally Invasive Esophagectomy) trial and showed that the minimally invasive approach has similar oncologic outcomes with lower complication rates, decreased perioperative morbidity, and better quality-of-life parameters. Although this was a small trial (59 patients in minimally invasive group vs 56 with open approach), the results were promising and favored minimally invasive surgery in the ongoing comparative debate on the optimal choice of operative approaches.[95]

Another area of debate is the extent of lymphadenectomy. Lymphadenectomy is performed to achieve 2 objectives: accurate staging and providing a potential survival benefit by removing locally advanced disease. In general, Eastern surgeons advocate for more extensive lymphadenectomy compared with their Western counterparts. Extended lymphadenectomy performed as a complete 3-field or 2-field lymphadenectomy is more commonly practiced in Eastern countries, especially Japan, but is performed in few institutions in the Western hemisphere.[96] Most Western institutions perform a limited 2-field lymphadenectomy. These differences are driven by multiple factors, including variation in predominant histologic subtypes, location of tumor, and neoadjuvant treatment effect. Because SCC is the predominant histology in Eastern countries, and SCC tumors are frequently located more proximally than the AC tumors, cervical, mediastinal, and abdominal lymph nodes can be involved at various frequencies.[97] Therefore, adequate staging of SCC may require complete 3-field or 2-field lymphadenectomy.

Investigators also question the effect of neoadjuvant chemotherapy or chemoradiation therapy on lymph node involvement. Because chemoradiation therapy is more often used in Western countries, many Western surgeons have found that lymph nodes are often difficult to find after treatment and question whether an extended lymph node is possible or even necessary. To investigate this association, Koen Talsma and colleagues[98] studied the cohort of patients enrolled in the CROSS trial and showed a direct correlation between the total number of resected lymph nodes and overall survival among patients in the esophagectomy-only arm. However, this association was not present in the group having neoadjuvant treatment followed by surgery. The presence of extensive lymphadenopathy was accordingly questioned in patients who received neoadjuvant chemoradiation because the absence of involved lymph nodes may be caused by the sterilizing effect of neoadjuvant treatment, and, therefore, accurate staging by lymphadenectomy is not possible. Nonetheless, in Western countries, there are no clear guidelines for the extent of lymphadenectomy, although it is established that at least 15 lymph nodes should be harvested to achieve optimal oncologic outcomes.[99] In order to standardize lymphadenectomy in Western countries, a multicenter prospective trial (the TIGER study: ClinicalTrials.gov identifier: NCT03222895) is designed to identify the location of lymph node metastases. This information may provide evidence-based guidelines for standardizing lymphadenectomy in the Western population.

MOLECULAR LANDSCAPE, GROUND ZERO OF HETEROGENEITY IN TREATMENT RESPONSE?

Unraveling the molecular landscape of esophageal cancer is imperative for the better understanding of the disease pathogenesis and the discovery of diagnostic biomarkers and druggable therapeutic targets. In a comprehensive analysis of both Eastern and Western populations, The Cancer Genome Atlas (TCGA) Research Network has performed an integrated genomic characterization of esophageal cancer.[100] They were able to show a molecular separation between SCC and AC with lineage-specific changes driving tumor development toward either SCC or AC. The investigators showed that certain signal transduction pathways, such as p63 (squamous epithelial differentiation), Wnt, and syndecan, were overexpressed in SCC, whereas FOXA and ARF6-dependent E-cadherin signaling and E-cadherin–regulating pathways played a more significant role in AC tumorigenesis. In addition, the molecular landscape of SCC was more similar to the molecular landscape of SCC of other organs than that of AC. SCC was classified into 3 molecular subtypes with distinct molecular alterations and biological consequences. Frequent genetic alterations were observed in CCND1, SOX2, and TP63. However, AC more closely resembled gastric AC and was distinct from SCC with frequent genomic amplifications identified in ERBB2, VEGFA, and GATA4 and GATA6. These significant contrasts support the idea that the two subtypes should be separated in both research studies and therapeutic approaches.[100]

SCC molecular subtypes are designated esophageal SCC (ESCC) 1, ESCC2, and ESCC3 with trends for geographic associations from the TCGA study. In their study cohort, patients with Asian background tended to have ESCC1, characterized by alterations in NRF2 pathways, which are important against oxidative damage from various insults such as carcinogens and chemotherapy agents. NRF2 mutations have been reported to confer resistance to systemic therapy in various malignancies, including esophageal cancer.[101–103] The ESCC2 subtype was more frequently observed in patients from Eastern Europe and South America, and all patients with ESCC3 (total of 4) were from North America (United States and Canada). Trends in geographic association found in the TCGA study need to be further investigated in larger study populations. The results of this study also corroborated the findings of previously published reports showing molecular distinction between SCC and AC.[104] In another comprehensive comparative genomic analysis of SCC and AC, Lin and colleagues[105] aggregated mutational profiles of 1048 patients with esophageal cancer from TCGA and the International Cancer Genome Consortium. Differences between SCC and AC in subtype-specific mutational signatures and mutually exclusive sets of driver genes, including 9 novel subtype-specific significantly mutated genes, provide further evidence that there is a sharp contrast between SCC and AC at the molecular level. These findings strongly support the notion that therapeutic approaches for esophageal SCC and AC should be treated as separate entities, particularly in clinical trials.

Although comparative epidemiology of esophageal SCC and AC has been extensively studied, geographic variations of molecular alterations in esophageal cancer have not been as widely investigated. In a study from the California Cancer Registry, Kim and colleagues[106] showed that the incidence of SCC was higher in all Asians, whether born in the United States or abroad, compared with non-Hispanic white people. There were also significant variations in the incidence of esophageal cancer among Asian ethnicities. Foreign-born Japanese and Vietnamese had the highest incidence of SCC. In contrast, the incidence of AC was uniformly lower in all groups of Asians compared with non-Hispanic white people. The findings reciprocate the global patterns and consequentially emphasize the role of genetic factors in racial/ethnic variations in the development of esophageal cancer. Chen and colleagues[107] reported similar findings from the Surveillance, Epidemiology, and End Results (SEER) database. To further investigate the role of genetic factors in racial/ethnic differences, they performed a comparative analysis of genome-wide mutations, epigenetic alterations, and expression profiles of Asians versus white patients, obtained from Broad Genome Data Analysis Centers.[107] Although the global profiles were similar between white people and Asians, significant differences were also observed. Various genes from similar pathways harbored differential mutational changes. An example was the KEAP1-NRF2 pathway. Although KEAP1 alterations were observed to be significantly higher in white people, NRF2 mutations were more frequent in Asians. Both genes belong to a pathway that protects the cells against oxidative stress. At the epigenetic level, Asians have higher methylations of various genes, such as tissue factor pathway inhibitor (TFPI) or PIK3R1. The PIK3/AKT pathway plays a role in cancer progression and metastasis of SCC and is under investigation as a therapeutic target.[108] Correspondingly, the global gene expression levels were similar between Asians and white people, whereas 63 genes were identified to be differentially expressed. Among these were WNT and FZD9, which belong to the Wnt signaling pathway and are expressed significantly higher in Asians.

In an analysis of heritability based on genome-wide association studies (GWASs) of 13 different cancer types, SCC was shown to have the highest heritability.[109] GWASs from 3 Chinese studies and 1 European study have identified genetic variants that are associated with an increased risk of SCC carcinogenesis.[110,111] Smaller studies have investigated specific genetic variations and single nucleotide polymorphisms that increase the risk of SCC in association with known environmental risk factors such as tobacco use and alcohol consumption.[112,113] Various GWASs have also evaluated the susceptibility of specific genetic variations to AC and their associated increased risk of AC with Barrett esophagus. A large pooled analysis of all the previously published GWASs verified 8 previously reported and 8 newly identified risk gene loci. Although, to date, the clinical utility of these findings is limited, identification of genetic variants has enhanced knowledge about the influence of genetic factors in patients' susceptibilities to esophageal cancer and elucidated understanding of the esophageal carcinogenesis pathways. A growing body of evidence suggests that the differences in the molecular profiles of tumors from various geographic regions may contribute to the variations in the diagnostic and therapeutic outcomes. Further investigation to delineate the discrepancies in carcinogenic pathways and epigenetic mechanisms among divergent regions of the world is necessary to provide accurate treatment algorithms.

SUMMARY AND FUTURE DIRECTIONS

Esophageal cancer comprises 2 distinct histologic subtypes with distinct geographic variations, epidemiologic features, molecular profiles, and genetic signatures. These variations are the basis of diversity in clinicopathologic features of tumors and inconsistencies in management of this heterogeneous disease. Despite all the recent advancements, knowledge about the complex interplay between environmental factors, genetic susceptibilities, and subsequent molecular alterations leading to the development of esophageal cancer is limited. Identifying these complex interactions is the crucial step to design more specific and targeted therapeutic approaches.

Geographic variations of esophageal cancer have led to discrepancies in the management of this disease across the world. Treatment strategies have been more standardized in Western countries. Except for in situ or early-stage disease, which can be managed with esophagectomy alone or endoscopic resections, multimodality therapy with neoadjuvant chemoradiation followed by esophagectomy is widely accepted based on high-level evidence. Definitive chemoradiation is an acceptable alternative in patients who are not surgical candidates or patients who wish to avoid surgery. Although salvage therapy is a viable option, long-term outcomes are unclear, but it can be considered in select patients. However, in Eastern countries, these results have not been widely accepted or validated. Nevertheless, there is a paradigm shift toward neoadjuvant chemoradiation followed by esophagectomy in some Eastern countries, and in others, like Japan, neoadjuvant chemotherapy has become the current standard of care. Ongoing trials are investigating neoadjuvant chemoradiation. These results will shape the therapeutic multimodality approach in the near future. Multiple surgical approaches are currently practiced for esophagectomy, and although minor variations exist, dependent on tumor location and surgeon preference, no single approach has been shown to be superior. Minimally invasive esophagectomy is an acceptable surgical option with equivalent oncologic outcomes and superior patient satisfaction. Lymphadenectomy is more standardized in Eastern countries, whereas Western surgeons often elect to modify the extent of lymphadenectomy based on the patient's clinical features. An ongoing Western prospective study investigating patterns of lymph node involvement will provide key information as to how best to standardize lymphadenectomy.

There exists a wide variation in treatment response for patients with esophageal cancer. Further prospective studies and randomized trials are necessary to address these variations. The many studies indicating divergent genetic evolution of esophageal cancer between Eastern and Western populations have shown the importance of the molecular landscape in determining appropriate treatment algorithms. By integrating molecular profiling as part of the management of patients with esophageal cancer, future treatment guidelines will provide a more personalized and effective approach to this disease.

REFERENCES

1. Dubecz A, Schwartz SI. Franz John A. Torek. Ann Thorac Surg 2008;85(4): 1497–9.
2. Ferlay J, Soerjomataram I, Dikshit R, et al. Cancer incidence and mortality worldwide: sources, methods and major patterns in GLOBOCAN 2012. Int J Cancer 2015;136(5):E359–86.

3. Esophageal cancer: epidemiology, pathogenesis and prevention. Nat Clin Pract Gastroenterol Hepatol 2008;5(9):517–26.

4. Coleman HG, Xie SH, Lagergren J. The epidemiology of esophageal adenocarcinoma. Gastroenterology 2018;154(2):390–405.

5. Spechler SJ. Barrett esophagus and risk of esophageal cancer: a clinical review. JAMA 2013;310(6):627–36.

6. Engel LS, Chow WH, Vaughan TL, et al. Population attributable risks of esophageal and gastric cancers. J Natl Cancer Inst 2003;95(18):1404–13.

7. Tran GD, Sun XD, Abnet CC, et al. Prospective study of risk factors for esophageal and gastric cancers in the Linxian general population trial cohort in China. Int J Cancer 2005;113(3):456–63.

8. Abnet CC, Arnold M, Wei WQ. Epidemiology of esophageal squamous cell carcinoma. Gastroenterology 2018;154(2):360–73.

9. Freedman ND, Abnet CC, Leitzmann MF, et al. A prospective study of tobacco, alcohol, and the risk of esophageal and gastric cancer subtypes. Am J Epidemiol 2007;165(12):1424–33.

10. Zendehdel K, Nyren O, Luo J, et al. Risk of gastroesophageal cancer among smokers and users of Scandinavian moist snuff. Int J Cancer 2008;122(5): 1095–9.

11. Ishiguro S, Sasazuki S, Inoue M, et al. Effect of alcohol consumption, cigarette smoking and flushing response on esophageal cancer risk: a population-based cohort study (JPHC study). Cancer Lett 2009;275(2):240–6.

12. Nasrollahzadeh D, Kamangar F, Aghcheli K, et al. Opium, tobacco, and alcohol use in relation to oesophageal squamous cell carcinoma in a high-risk area of Iran. Br J Cancer 2008;98(11):1857–63.

13. Wang JB, Fan JH, Liang H, et al. Attributable causes of esophageal cancer incidence and mortality in China. PLoS One 2012;7(8):e42281.

14. Gao Y, Hu N, Han XY, et al. Risk factors for esophageal and gastric cancers in Shanxi Province, China: a case-control study. Cancer Epidemiol 2011;35(6): e91–9.

15. Lubin JH, De Stefani E, Abnet CC, et al. Mate drinking and esophageal squamous cell carcinoma in South America: pooled results from two large multicenter case-control studies. Cancer Epidemiol Biomarkers Prev 2014;23(1):107–16.

16. Islami F, Pourshams A, Nasrollahzadeh D, et al. Tea drinking habits and oesophageal cancer in a high risk area in northern Iran: population based case-control study. BMJ 2009;338:b929.

17. Loomis D, Guyton KZ, Grosse Y, et al. Carcinogenicity of drinking coffee, mate, and very hot beverages. Lancet Oncol 2016;17(7):877–8.

18. Murphy G, McCormack V, Abedi-Ardekani B, et al. International cancer seminars: a focus on esophageal squamous cell carcinoma. Ann Oncol 2017; 28(9):2086–93.

19. Cook MB, Corley DA, Murray LJ, et al. Gastroesophageal reflux in relation to adenocarcinomas of the esophagus: a pooled analysis from the Barrett's and Esophageal Adenocarcinoma Consortium (BEACON). PLoS One 2014;9(7): e103508.

20. Drahos J, Xiao Q, Risch HA, et al. Age-specific risk factor profiles of adenocarcinomas of the esophagus: a pooled analysis from the international BEACON consortium. Int J Cancer 2016;138(1):55–64.

21. Shiota S, Singh S, Anshasi A, et al. Prevalence of Barrett's esophagus in Asian countries: a systematic review and meta-analysis. Clin Gastroenterol Hepatol 2015;13(11):1907–18.

22. Whiteman DC, Sadeghi S, Pandeya N, et al. Combined effects of obesity, acid reflux and smoking on the risk of adenocarcinomas of the oesophagus. Gut 2008;57(2):173–80.

23. Lagergren J, Bergstrom R, Nyren O. Association between body mass and adenocarcinoma of the esophagus and gastric cardia. Ann Intern Med 1999; 130(11):883–90.

24. Cook MB, Kamangar F, Whiteman DC, et al. Cigarette smoking and adenocarcinomas of the esophagus and esophagogastric junction: a pooled analysis from the international BEACON consortium. J Natl Cancer Inst 2010;102(17): 1344–53.

25. Wang QL, Xie SH, Li WT, et al. Smoking cessation and risk of esophageal cancer by histological type: systematic review and meta-analysis. J Natl Cancer Inst 2017;109(12).

26. Freedman ND, Murray LJ, Kamangar F, et al. Alcohol intake and risk of oesophageal adenocarcinoma: a pooled analysis from the BEACON Consortium. Gut 2011;60(8):1029–37.

27. Wang M, Gu XZ, Yin WB, et al. Randomized clinical trial on the combination of preoperative irradiation and surgery in the treatment of esophageal carcinoma: report on 206 patients. Int J Radiat Oncol Biol Phys 1989;16(2):325–7.

28. Gignoux M, Roussel A, Paillot B, et al. The value of preoperative radiotherapy in esophageal cancer: results of a study by the EORTC. Recent Results Cancer Res 1988;110:1–13.

29. Maipang T, Vasinanukorn P, Petpichetchian C, et al. Induction chemotherapy in the treatment of patients with carcinoma of the esophagus. J Surg Oncol 1994; 56(3):191–7.

30. Baba M, Natsugoe S, Shimada M, et al. Prospective evaluation of preoperative chemotherapy in resectable squamous cell carcinoma of the thoracic esophagus. Dis Esophagus 2000;13(2):136–41.

31. Wang C, Ding T, Chang L. A randomized clinical study of preoperative chemotherapy for esophageal carcinoma. Zhonghua Zhong Liu Za Zhi 2001;23(3): 254–5 [in Chinese].

32. Ando N, Kato H, Igaki H, et al. A randomized trial comparing postoperative adjuvant chemotherapy with cisplatin and 5-fluorouracil versus preoperative chemotherapy for localized advanced squamous cell carcinoma of the thoracic esophagus (JCOG9907). Ann Surg Oncol 2012;19(1):68–74.

33. Zheng Y, Li Y, Liu X, et al. Reevaluation of neoadjuvant chemotherapy for esophageal squamous cell carcinoma: a meta-analysis of randomized controlled trials over the past 20 years. Medicine (Baltimore) 2015;94(27):e1102.

34. An FS, Huang JQ, Xie YT, et al. A prospective study of combined chemoradiotherapy followed by surgery in the treatment of esophageal carcinoma. Zhonghua Zhong Liu Za Zhi 2003;25(4):376–9 [in Chinese].

35. Cao XF, He XT, Ji L, et al. Effects of neoadjuvant radiochemotherapy on pathological staging and prognosis for locally advanced esophageal squamous cell carcinoma. Dis Esophagus 2009;22(6):477–81.

36. Lee JL, Park SI, Kim SB, et al. A single institutional phase III trial of preoperative chemotherapy with hyperfractionation radiotherapy plus surgery versus surgery alone for resectable esophageal squamous cell carcinoma. Ann Oncol 2004; 15(6):947–54.

37. Natsugoe S, Okumura H, Matsumoto M, et al. Randomized controlled study on preoperative chemoradiotherapy followed by surgery versus surgery alone for

esophageal squamous cell cancer in a single institution. Dis Esophagus 2006; 19(6):468–72.

38. Yang H, Liu H, Chen Y, et al. Neoadjuvant chemoradiotherapy followed by surgery versus surgery alone for locally advanced squamous cell carcinoma of the esophagus (NEOCRTEC5010): a phase III multicenter, randomized, open-label clinical trial. J Clin Oncol 2018;36(27):2796–803.

39. Doosti-Irani A, Holakouie-Naieni K, Rahimi-Foroushani A, et al. A network meta-analysis of the treatments for esophageal squamous cell carcinoma in terms of survival. Crit Rev Oncol Hematol 2018;127:80–90.

40. Nakamura K, Kato K, Igaki H, et al. Three-arm phase III trial comparing cisplatin plus 5-FU (CF) versus docetaxel, cisplatin plus 5-FU (DCF) versus radiotherapy with CF (CF-RT) as preoperative therapy for locally advanced esophageal cancer (JCOG1109, NExT study). Jpn J Clin Oncol 2013;43(7):752–5.

41. Fok M, Sham JS, Choy D, et al. Postoperative radiotherapy for carcinoma of the esophagus: a prospective, randomized controlled study. Surgery 1993;113(2):138–47.

42. Xiao ZF, Yang ZY, Liang J, et al. Value of radiotherapy after radical surgery for esophageal carcinoma: a report of 495 patients. Ann Thorac Surg 2003;75(2):331–6.

43. Teniere P, Hay JM, Fingerhut A, et al. Postoperative radiation therapy does not increase survival after curative resection for squamous cell carcinoma of the middle and lower esophagus as shown by a multicenter controlled trial. French University Association for Surgical Research. Surg Gynecol Obstet 1991;173(2):123–30.

44. Zieren HU, Muller JM, Jacobi CA, et al. Adjuvant postoperative radiation therapy after curative resection of squamous cell carcinoma of the thoracic esophagus: a prospective randomized study. World J Surg 1995;19(3):444–9.

45. Ando N, Iizuka T, Ide H, et al. Surgery plus chemotherapy compared with surgery alone for localized squamous cell carcinoma of the thoracic esophagus: a Japan Clinical Oncology Group Study–JCOG9204. J Clin Oncol 2003;21(24):4592–6.

46. Tanaka Y, Yoshida K, Suetsugu T, et al. Recent advancements in esophageal cancer treatment in Japan. Ann Gastroenterol Surg 2018;2(4):253–65.

47. Hironaka S, Ohtsu A, Boku N, et al. Nonrandomized comparison between definitive chemoradiotherapy and radical surgery in patients with T(2-3)N(any) M(0) squamous cell carcinoma of the esophagus. Int J Radiat Oncol Biol Phys 2003;57(2):425–33.

48. Toh Y, Ohga T, Itoh S, et al. Treatment results of radical surgery and definitive chemoradiotherapy for patients with submucosal esophageal squamous cell cancinomas. Anticancer Res 2006;26(3B):2487–91.

49. Yamashita H, Okuma K, Seto Y, et al. A retrospective comparison of clinical outcomes and quality of life measures between definitive chemoradiation alone and radical surgery for clinical stage II-III esophageal carcinoma. J Surg Oncol 2009;100(6):435–41.

50. Yamashita H, Nakagawa K, Yamada K, et al. A single institutional non-randomized retrospective comparison between definitive chemoradiotherapy and radical surgery in 82 Japanese patients with resectable esophageal squamous cell carcinoma. Dis Esophagus 2008;21(5):430–6.

51. Ariga H, Nemoto K, Miyazaki S, et al. Prospective comparison of surgery alone and chemoradiotherapy with selective surgery in resectable squamous cell carcinoma of the esophagus. Int J Radiat Oncol Biol Phys 2009;75(2):348–56.

52. Yamamoto S, Ishihara R, Motoori M, et al. Comparison between definitive che-moradiotherapy and esophagectomy in patients with clinical stage I esophageal squamous cell carcinoma. Am J Gastroenterol 2011;106(6):1048–54.

53. Motoori M, Yano M, Ishihara R, et al. Comparison between radical esophagec-tomy and definitive chemoradiotherapy in patients with clinical T1bN0M0 esoph-ageal cancer. Ann Surg Oncol 2012;19(7):2135–41.

54. Park I, Kim YH, Yoon DH, et al. Non-surgical treatment versus radical esopha-gectomy for clinical T1N0M0 esophageal carcinoma: a single-center experi-ence. Cancer Chemother Pharmacol 2014;74(5):995–1003.

55. Matsuda S, Tsubosa Y, Niihara M, et al. Comparison of transthoracic esopha-gectomy with definitive chemoradiotherapy as initial treatment for patients with esophageal squamous cell carcinoma who could tolerate transthoracic esophagectomy. Ann Surg Oncol 2015;22(6):1866–73.

56. Teoh AY, Chiu PW, Yeung WK, et al. Long-term survival outcomes after definitive chemoradiation versus surgery in patients with resectable squamous carcinoma of the esophagus: results from a randomized controlled trial. Ann Oncol 2013; 24(1):165–71.

57. Ma MW, Gao XS, Gu XB, et al. The role of definitive chemoradiotherapy versus surgery as initial treatments for potentially resectable esophageal carcinoma. World J Surg Oncol 2018;16(1):172.

58. Kato K, Muro K, Minashi K, et al. Phase II study of chemoradiotherapy with 5-fluorouracil and cisplatin for Stage II-III esophageal squamous cell carcinoma: JCOG trial (JCOG 9906). Int J Radiat Oncol Biol Phys 2011;81(3):684–90.

59. Kato H, Sato A, Fukuda H, et al. A phase II trial of chemoradiotherapy for stage I esophageal squamous cell carcinoma: Japan Clinical Oncology Group Study (JCOG9708). Jpn J Clin Oncol 2009;39(10):638–43.

60. Sohda M, Kuwano H. Current status and future prospects for esophageal can-cer treatment. Ann Thorac Cardiovasc Surg 2017;23(1):1–11.

61. Nishimura M, Daiko H, Yoshida J, et al. Salvage esophagectomy following defin-itive chemoradiotherapy. Gen Thorac Cardiovasc Surg 2007;55(11):461–4 [dis-cussion: 464–5].

62. Kumagai K, Mariosa D, Tsai JA, et al. Systematic review and meta-analysis on the significance of salvage esophagectomy for persistent or recurrent esopha-geal squamous cell carcinoma after definitive chemoradiotherapy. Dis Esoph-agus 2016;29(7):734–9.

63. Arnott SJ, Duncan W, Kerr GR, et al. Low dose preoperative radiotherapy for carcinoma of the oesophagus: results of a randomized clinical trial. Radiother Oncol 1992;24(2):108–13.

64. Launois B, Delarue D, Campion JP, et al. Preoperative radiotherapy for carci-noma of the esophagus. Surg Gynecol Obstet 1981;153(5):690–2.

65. Arnott SJ, Duncan W, Gignoux M, et al. Preoperative radiotherapy in esophageal carcinoma: a meta-analysis using individual patient data (Oesophageal Cancer Collaborative Group). Int J Radiat Oncol Biol Phys 1998;41(3):579–83.

66. Herskovic A, Martz K, al-Sarraf M, et al. Combined chemotherapy and radio-therapy compared with radiotherapy alone in patients with cancer of the esoph-agus. N Engl J Med 1992;326(24):1593–8.

67. Roth JA, Pass HI, Flanagan MM, et al. Randomized clinical trial of preoperative and postoperative adjuvant chemotherapy with cisplatin, vindesine, and bleo-mycin for carcinoma of the esophagus. J Thorac Cardiovasc Surg 1988;96(2): 242–8.

68. Schlag PM. Randomized trial of preoperative chemotherapy for squamous cell cancer of the esophagus. The Chirurgische Arbeitsgemeinschaft Fuer Onkologie der Deutschen Gesellschaft Fuer Chirurgie Study Group. Arch Surg 1992; 127(12):1446-50.

69. Ancona E, Ruol A, Santi S, et al. Only pathologic complete response to neoadjuvant chemotherapy improves significantly the long term survival of patients with resectable esophageal squamous cell carcinoma: final report of a randomized, controlled trial of preoperative chemotherapy versus surgery alone. Cancer 2001;91(11):2165-74.

70. Medical Research Council Oesophageal Cancer Working Group. Surgical resection with or without preoperative chemotherapy in oesophageal cancer: a randomised controlled trial. Lancet 2002;359(9319):1727-33.

71. Allum WH, Stenning SP, Bancewicz J, et al. Long-term results of a randomized trial of surgery with or without preoperative chemotherapy in esophageal cancer. J Clin Oncol 2009;27(30):5062-7.

72. Bhansali MS, Vaidya JS, Bhatt RG, et al. Chemotherapy for carcinoma of the esophagus: a comparison of evidence from meta-analyses of randomized trials and of historical control studies. Ann Oncol 1996;7(4):355-9.

73. Urschel JD, Vasan H, Blewett CJ. A meta-analysis of randomized controlled trials that compared neoadjuvant chemotherapy and surgery to surgery alone for resectable esophageal cancer. Am J Surg 2002;183(3):274-9.

74. Malthaner R, Fenlon D. Preoperative chemotherapy for resectable thoracic esophageal cancer. Cochrane Database Syst Rev 2003;(4):CD001556.

75. Kidane B, Coughlin S, Vogt K, et al. Preoperative chemotherapy for resectable thoracic esophageal cancer. Cochrane Database Syst Rev 2015;(5):CD001556.

76. Kelsen DP, Ginsberg R, Pajak TF, et al. Chemotherapy followed by surgery compared with surgery alone for localized esophageal cancer. N Engl J Med 1998;339(27):1979-84.

77. Cunningham D, Allum WH, Stenning SP, et al. Perioperative chemotherapy versus surgery alone for resectable gastroesophageal cancer. N Engl J Med 2006;355(1):11-20.

78. van Hagen P, Hulshof MC, van Lanschot JJ, et al. Preoperative chemoradiotherapy for esophageal or junctional cancer. N Engl J Med 2012;366(22):2074-84.

79. Shapiro J, van Lanschot JJB, Hulshof M, et al. Neoadjuvant chemoradiotherapy plus surgery versus surgery alone for oesophageal or junctional cancer (CROSS): long-term results of a randomised controlled trial. Lancet Oncol 2015;16(9):1090-8.

80. Toxopeus E, van der Schaaf M, van Lanschot J, et al. Outcome of patients treated within and outside a randomized clinical trial on neoadjuvant chemoradiotherapy plus surgery for esophageal cancer: extrapolation of a randomized clinical trial (CROSS). Ann Surg Oncol 2018;25(8):2441-8.

81. Ychou M, Boige V, Pignon JP, et al. Perioperative chemotherapy compared with surgery alone for resectable gastroesophageal adenocarcinoma: an FNCLCC and FFCD multicenter phase III trial. J Clin Oncol 2011;29(13):1715-21.

82. Pouliquen X, Levard H, Hay JM, et al. 5-Fluorouracil and cisplatin therapy after palliative surgical resection of squamous cell carcinoma of the esophagus. A multicenter randomized trial. French Associations for Surgical Research. Ann Surg 1996;223(2):127-33.

83. Cooper JS, Guo MD, Herskovic A, et al. Chemoradiotherapy of locally advanced esophageal cancer: long-term follow-up of a prospective randomized trial

(RTOG 85-01). Radiation Therapy Oncology Group. JAMA 1999;281(17): 1623–7.

84. Minsky BD, Pajak TF, Ginsberg RJ, et al. INT 0123 (Radiation Therapy Oncology Group 94-05) phase III trial of combined-modality therapy for esophageal cancer: high-dose versus standard-dose radiation therapy. J Clin Oncol 2002;20(5): 1167–74.

85. Bedenne L, Michel P, Bouche O, et al. Chemoradiation followed by surgery compared with chemoradiation alone in squamous cancer of the esophagus: FFCD 9102. J Clin Oncol 2007;25(10):1160–8.

86. Swisher SG, Moughan J, Komaki RU, et al. Final results of NRG oncology RTOG 0246: an organ-preserving selective resection strategy in esophageal cancer patients treated with definitive chemoradiation. J Thorac Oncol 2017;12(2): 368–74.

87. Barreto JC, Posner MC. Transhiatal versus transthoracic esophagectomy for esophageal cancer. World J Gastroenterol 2010;16(30):3804–10.

88. Goldminc M, Maddern G, Le Prise E, et al. Oesophagectomy by a transhiatal approach or thoracotomy: a prospective randomized trial. Br J Surg 1993; 80(3):367–70.

89. Chu KM, Law SY, Fok M, et al. A prospective randomized comparison of transhiatal and transthoracic resection for lower-third esophageal carcinoma. Am J Surg 1997;174(3):320–4.

90. Jacobi CA, Zieren HU, Muller JM, et al. Surgical therapy of esophageal carcinoma: the influence of surgical approach and esophageal resection on cardiopulmonary function. Eur J Cardiothorac Surg 1997;11(1):32–7.

91. Hulscher JB, van Sandick JW, de Boer AG, et al. Extended transthoracic resection compared with limited transhiatal resection for adenocarcinoma of the esophagus. N Engl J Med 2002;347(21):1662–9.

92. Hulscher JB, Tijssen JG, Obertop H, et al. Transthoracic versus transhiatal resection for carcinoma of the esophagus: a meta-analysis. Ann Thorac Surg 2001;72(1):306–13.

93. Shaikh T, Meyer JE, Horwitz EM. Optimal use of combined modality therapy in the treatment of esophageal cancer. Surg Oncol Clin N Am 2017;26(3):405–29.

94. Straatman J, van der Wielen N, Cuesta MA, et al. Minimally invasive versus open esophageal resection: three-year follow-up of the previously reported randomized controlled trial: the TIME trial. Ann Surg 2017;266(2):232–6.

95. Tan L, Tang H. Oncological outcomes of the TIME trial in esophageal cancer: is it the era of minimally invasive esophagectomy? Ann Transl Med 2018;6(4):85.

96. Pennathur A, Luketich JD. Resection for esophageal cancer: strategies for optimal management. Ann Thorac Surg 2008;85(2):S751–6.

97. Akiyama H, Tsurumaru M, Udagawa H, et al. Radical lymph node dissection for cancer of the thoracic esophagus. Ann Surg 1994;220(3):364–72 [discussion: 372–3].

98. Koen Talsma A, Shapiro J, Looman CW, et al. Lymph node retrieval during esophagectomy with and without neoadjuvant chemoradiotherapy: prognostic and therapeutic impact on survival. Ann Surg 2014;260(5):786–92 [discussion: 792–3].

99. Hagens ERC, van Berge Henegouwen MI, Cuesta MA, et al. The extent of lymphadenectomy in esophageal resection for cancer should be standardized. J Thorac Dis 2017;9(Suppl 8):S713–23.

100. Cancer Genome Atlas Research Network, Analysis Working Group: Asan University, BC Cancer Agency, et al. Integrated genomic characterization of oesophageal carcinoma. Nature 2017;541(7636):169–75.

101. Shibata T, Kokubu A, Saito S, et al. NRF2 mutation confers malignant potential and resistance to chemoradiation therapy in advanced esophageal squamous cancer. Neoplasia 2011;13(9):864–73.

102. Karathedath S, Rajamani BM, Musheer Aalam SM, et al. Role of NF-E2 related factor 2 (Nrf2) on chemotherapy resistance in acute myeloid leukemia (AML) and the effect of pharmacological inhibition of Nrf2. PLoS One 2017;12(5): e0177227.

103. Bai X, Chen Y, Hou X, et al. Emerging role of NRF2 in chemoresistance by regulating drug-metabolizing enzymes and efflux transporters. Drug Metab Rev 2016;48(4):541–67.

104. Wang K, Johnson A, Ali SM, et al. Comprehensive genomic profiling of advanced esophageal squamous cell carcinomas and esophageal adenocarcinomas reveals similarities and differences. Oncologist 2015;20(10):1132–9.

105. Lin DC, Dinh HQ, Xie JJ, et al. Identification of distinct mutational patterns and new driver genes in oesophageal squamous cell carcinomas and adenocarcinomas. Gut 2018;67(10):1769–79.

106. Kim JY, Winters JK, Kim J, et al. Birthplace and esophageal cancer incidence patterns among Asian-Americans. Dis Esophagus 2016;29(1):99–104.

107. Chen S, Zhou K, Yang L, et al. Racial differences in esophageal squamous cell carcinoma: incidence and molecular features. Biomed Res Int 2017;2017: 1204082.

108. Li B, Xu WW, Lam AKY, et al. Significance of PI3K/AKT signaling pathway in metastasis of esophageal squamous cell carcinoma and its potential as a target for anti-metastasis therapy. Oncotarget 2017;8(24):38755–66.

109. Sampson JN, Wheeler WA, Yeager M, et al. Analysis of heritability and shared heritability based on genome-wide association studies for thirteen cancer types. J Natl Cancer Inst 2015;107(12):djv279.

110. Wu C, Wang Z, Song X, et al. Joint analysis of three genome-wide association studies of esophageal squamous cell carcinoma in Chinese populations. Nat Genet 2014;46(9):1001–6.

111. McKay JD, Truong T, Gaborieau V, et al. A genome-wide association study of upper aerodigestive tract cancers conducted within the INHANCE consortium. PLoS Genet 2011;7(3):e1001333.

112. Moaven O, Raziee HR, Sima HR, et al. Interactions between Glutathione-S-Transferase M1, T1 and P1 polymorphisms and smoking, and increased susceptibility to esophageal squamous cell carcinoma. Cancer Epidemiol 2010; 34(3):285–90.

113. Yokoyama T, Yokoyama A, Kato H, et al. Alcohol flushing, alcohol and aldehyde dehydrogenase genotypes, and risk for esophageal squamous cell carcinoma in Japanese men. Cancer Epidemiol Biomarkers Prev 2003;12(11 Pt 1): 1227–33.

114. Apinop C, Puttisak P, Preecha N. A prospective study of combined therapy in esophageal cancer. Hepatogastroenterology 1994;41(4):391–3.

115. Nygaard K, Hagen S, Hansen HS, et al. Pre-operative radiotherapy prolongs survival in operable esophageal carcinoma: a randomized, multicenter study of pre-operative radiotherapy and chemotherapy. The second Scandinavian trial in esophageal cancer. World J Surg 1992;16(6):1104–9 [discussion: 1110].

116. Le Prise E, Etienne PL, Meunier B, et al. A randomized study of chemotherapy, radiation therapy, and surgery versus surgery for localized squamous cell carcinoma of the esophagus. Cancer 1994;73(7):1779–84.

117. Walsh TN, Noonan N, Hollywood D, et al. A comparison of multimodal therapy and surgery for esophageal adenocarcinoma. N Engl J Med 1996;335(7):462–7.

118. Bosset JF, Gignoux M, Triboulet JP, et al. Chemoradiotherapy followed by surgery compared with surgery alone in squamous-cell cancer of the esophagus. N Engl J Med 1997;337(3):161–7.

119. Urba SG, Orringer MB, Turrisi A, et al. Randomized trial of preoperative chemoradiation versus surgery alone in patients with locoregional esophageal carcinoma. J Clin Oncol 2001;19(2):305–13.

120. Tepper J, Krasna MJ, Niedzwiecki D, et al. Phase III trial of trimodality therapy with cisplatin, fluorouracil, radiotherapy, and surgery compared with surgery alone for esophageal cancer: CALGB 9781. J Clin Oncol 2008;26(7):1086–92.

Complications After Esophagectomy

Igor Wanko Mboumi, MD[a], Sushanth Reddy, MD[b], Anne O. Lidor, MD, MPH[a],*

KEYWORDS

- Esophageal leak • Esophageal stricture • Aspiration • Chylothorax • Feeding access

KEY POINTS

- Anastomotic leaks have a variety of presentations and should be considered in any patient with altered postoperative course.
- Wide drainage and establishing enteral nutritional access is the mainstay for treating anastomotic leaks.
- Cardiac arrhythmia corresponds to poor outcome after surgery and is often associated with pulmonary issues.
- Later complications are being increasingly reported after esophagectomy and include anastomotic stricture, delayed gastric emptying, and reflux.

INTRODUCTION

Esophageal cancer remains a worldwide health issue and is the eighth most common cancer throughout the globe.[1] Survival from this devastating disease is constantly improving with multimodal therapy. However, the key step in treating patients with esophageal cancer is surgical removal of the esophagus. Since its introduction by Czerny in the 1870s, esophagectomy has been feared for devastating postoperative outcomes. The mortality rates after esophagectomy have been steadily declining from a peak of 72% in the 1940s to 29% in the 1970s, 13% in the 1980s, and 9% in the 1990s.[2] Recent reviews demonstrate improved, yet formidable, modern 30-day and 90-day mortality rates of 2.4% and 4.5%, respectively. However, greater than half of all patients will still experience a complication.[3] Despite advances in technology and the development of operative techniques, the surgical treatment of the esophagus remains a challenge.

The authors have nothing to disclose.
[a] Division of Minimally Invasive and Bariatric Surgery, Department of Surgery, University of Wisconsin School of Medicine, 600 Highland Avenue K4/752, Madison, WI 53792-7375, USA;
[b] Department of Surgery, School of Medicine, The University of Alabama at Birmingham, Birmingham, AL 35294, USA
* Corresponding author.
E-mail address: lidor@surgery.wisc.edu

Surg Clin N Am 99 (2019) 501–510
https://doi.org/10.1016/j.suc.2019.02.011

Once the decision to perform an esophagectomy has been made, the decision on how to proceed must be made. The final decision can be based on surgeon comfort, experience, or patient-dependent factors. However, as in many aspects of surgery, the question of which technique(s) to use (trans-hiatal, Ivor-Lewis, 3-field techniques), what type of anastomosis (cervical or thoracic), or what type of approach (open, robotic, or laparoscopic/thoracoscopic) can be intimately linked to individual complications. Our objective is to outline and discuss some of the most common complications associated with esophagectomies and describe modern treatment approaches to overcome them. Complications still occur in 50% to 75% of all patients,[4–6] and the ability to care for and salvage these patients is paramount. This review focuses on anastomotic complications, chyle leaks, and cardiopulmonary complications, and late complications, including functional disorders such as delayed gastric emptying, reflux disease, and the occurrence of hiatal hernia after esophagectomy, are discussed.

ANASTOMOTIC LEAK

The most dreaded complication is an anastomotic leak. Historically, anastomotic leaks were associated with increased mortality, but this is no longer true.[7] The sequelae associated with anastomotic leaks can be dependent on the approach. Thoracic anastomosis (including Ivor-Lewis esophagectomy and the Sweet procedure ;left thoracoabdominal approach]) typically has 3% to 12% leak rates[8–11] compared with 10% to 25% associated with cervical anastomosis.[12,13] There are also significant variations regarding the method of anastomosis: hand sewn, stapled, type of suture, shape of the anastomosis.[14] There is no one way to perform an esophagectomy, and the surgeon should remain flexible and adaptable, because the procedure of choice is often dictated by the pathology at hand. Consequently, the surgeon should be able to recognize and promptly deal with the potential anastomotic complication.

Mortality from esophageal leaks was reported to be as high as 71% as recently as the 1990s.[15] In the last 20 years, preoperative chemoradiation has become the standard in treating esophageal cancers. Several studies have noted that preoperative chemoradiation increases the risk of anastomotic leak because the radiated esophagus is not easily amenable to suture and stapling techniques.[16,17] The segmental nature of the esophageal blood supply is often tenuous, relying on communicating branches. Furthermore, the stomach is the most commonly used conduit and is reliant on the right gastroepiploic artery for its blood supply. This tenuous blood supply for both the esophagus and stomach leads to a propensity for tissue ischemia and often even necrosis, leading to leaks. Also, because of this limited blood supply, precise and scrupulous surgical technique is important for postoperative success. Despite these pitfalls, mortality from leak rates continues to decrease.[7]

Prompt recognition of a leak is crucial. Clinical presentation of an anastomotic leak can be variable. For instance, cervical anastomotic leak may be recognizable from clinically apparent saliva in a neck drain or a neck wound inflammation/collection. A thoracic anastomotic leak into the pleural cavity can lead to early and late pulmonary symptoms as in respiratory insufficiency to the more severe acute respiratory distress syndrome (ARDS). Leaks may also present as tachycardia, other cardiac arrhythmias, hemodynamic instability, and abdominal pain. There can often be a subtle decline in mentation; this can be difficult to recognize in this class of patient who are often older and in the critical care unit. These patients can be falsely diagnosed with intensive care unit (ICU) delirium, and thus, a low threshold for prompt investigation, and a high level of suspicion can aid in diagnosis. The best tests for anastomotic failures are water-soluble contrast agent esophagogram, computed tomography (CT) of the abdomen and pelvis, and endoscopy. Although endoscopy can be feared because of a suggested risk of exacerbating the anastomotic leak, studies have proven it to be safe even with maximal insufflation.[18] In addition, endoscopy can not only be diagnostic but also therapeutic, with self-expandable medal stents, stent over sponge therapy, overstitch, and other endoscopic modalities (see later discussion). A simple classification system for anastomotic leaks has been derived from Lerut and helps guide treatment.

Several different analyses have demonstrated that patients with esophageal cancer are malnourished before resection.[19–21] Many centers routinely place a feeding jejunostomy tube either before or during esophagectomy. This practice has come under some scrutiny.[22–24] However, for patients who do develop anastomotic leaks, early jejunal feeding does seem to improve the likelihood of survival from surgery.[7] The added stress from inflammation on top of recent surgery combined with poor nutrition before surgery likely places an emphasis on adequate nutrition to heal from a leak.

Clinically minor leaks are those that demonstrate contained contrast extravasation on radiographs. Typically, these do not require additional intervention. If a nasogastric tube was placed across the esophagogastric anastomosis at the time of surgery, it should be kept in place. Enteral nutrition should be initiated if instituted distal to the stomach by either jejunostomy tube or nasoenteral nutrition. Parenteral nutrition can be considered, but enteral nutrition has been consistently shown to be superior to the parenteral route.[25–27]

Clinically major leaks in the chest can represent a therapeutic challenge. Drainage with tube thoracostomy and source control is of utmost importance. Many investigators have advocated for an aggressive reoperative approach for source control, including tissue flap reinforcement of the defect with muscle, pleura, pericardium, or omentum.[13,28,29] However, this strategy is often limited by which muscles were spared during the operative approach for the initial resection. Endoscopic management of esophageal leaks has gained favor in recent years. Although limited by the size of the defect needed for closure, endoscopic stenting can adequately close many anastomotic leaks with success rates of more than 80%.[30] Other techniques include endoscopic clips (success 56%–100%) and endoluminal vacuum therapy (success 86%–100%).[31] Endoscopic techniques are performed in selected patients by experienced endoscopists. In our practice, we favor trying endoscopic stenting for smaller defects. If that is not possible, we tend to prefer rotational muscle flaps based on the latissimus dorsi or serratus anterior muscle when reoperating for clinically major esophageal anastomotic leaks.

Severe leaks associated with conduit necrosis need to be diagnosed quickly. Even with early recognition and treatment, mortality approaches 90%.[32] Thankfully, this complication is relatively rare.[33] Most surgeons advocate removal of the conduit when it cannot be salvaged and strong consideration for cervical esophagostomy with distal enteral feeding access.[32,33] Because most patients are clinically ill, it is not recommended to attempt immediate alternate reconstruction. Should the patient survive, he/she should be referred to an experienced esophageal surgeon to consider alternative conduits (including colonic and supercharged jejunal interposition grafts). These patients should also be thoroughly counseled on quality of life expectations.

AIRWAY-GASTRIC FISTULA

Although relatively rare, with an incidence of 0.3% to 1.9%, this complication remains important because of its potential to lead to fatality. It is fitting to discuss airway gastric fistulas immediately after discussing anastomotic leaks because this, along with gastric staple line leaks, are likely the most common cause of the development of a fistula, with local inflammation from enteric contents and saliva causing a process of localized necrosis that can erode into the airway. In the acute period, its occurrence is often related to tracheal injury or postoperative mediastinitis.[34] Another factor that may act as catalyst for the formation of these airway-gastric fistula is a tracheal injury either by way of direct injury or by devascularization during dissection. Moreover, some have suggested that the proximity of the gastric conduit staple to the tracheal may also be a cause of this complication as a result of chronic inflammation of the gastric staple line. There is also considerable literature upholding adjunctive and neo-adjunctive treatment such as radiation and chemotherapy as causes for gastric airway fistulas.[35] A typical presentation of patients with this ailment is typically "cough with oral intake and shortness of breath due to aspiration of gastric contents" as well recurrent aspiration pneumonias and sepsis. The mainstay of diagnosis is an esophagram along with endoscopy as an adjunct diagnosis and treatment. Although CT scans can be helpful, they cannot rule out the presence of a gastric airway fistula. Treatment of this is most commonly achieved endoscopically with stenting when technically feasible and available. Surgery is reserved when stenting is not possible, unavailable, or unsuccessful.

RECURRENT LARYNGEAL NERVE PALSY

Recurrent laryngeal nerve palsy (RLNP) can lead to significant morbidity and mortality. Patients can present with symptoms such as hoarseness, dyspnea aspiration, pulmonary deterioration as a result of an inability to adequately protect the airway, including pneumonia, ARDS. Surgeons must be aware of the possibility of asphyxiation with bilateral recurrent nerve injury. This injury can be caused by a multitude of mechanisms during esophagectomies; some of the most common processes for injury are direct thermal injury, stretching injuries, compression, or vascular compromise.

The incidence of this injury is multifactorial, can be a result of technical aspects of the surgery or the size or extent of the tumor or different variabilities with regard to the recurrent laryngeal nerve. A retrospective study of 451 patients demonstrated that RLNP was associated with a McKeown approach and significantly increased hospital length of stay. In a study of 451 patients, a multivariate analysis was performed for patients with RLNP to assess its association with pulmonary morbidity and long-term functional recovery.[36] The investigators noted that half of these injuries recovered over the course of 18 months, suggesting that conservative management is sufficient for these patients.

CHYLE LEAKS

Chyle leaks are usually from a thoracic duct injury. This can especially be problematic in cases of mid-esophageal lesions or in surgical fields with scarring or distorted planes. The risk is greater in transthoracic approaches compared with transhiatal ones and is reported in 4% to 10% of cases. Chyle leaks can present as newly apparent pleural effusion; the fluid is often brown, white, or milky.[14] The diagnosis is made through fluid triglyceride analysis. Moreover, lymphoscintigraphy has been used to make the diagnosis with significant accuracy.[37] Most thoracic duct leaks will resolve with conservative management.[38] Nutrition is commonly altered to either total parenteral nutrition or a medium-chain triglyceride enteral formula.

Even when well drained, chyle leaks can result in significant comorbidities such as immunodeficiency, electrolyte imbalance, and malnutrition, with mortality rates reported from 10% to 50% in historical series.[39] Intervention is occasionally needed for chyle leaks. Patients with high output (with daily output >1 L) or persistent/prolonged (>2–4 weeks) leaks should be considered for an intervention. Most favor embolization of the thoracic duct with success rates reported in small retrospective series of 86% to 100%.[40,41] Surgical ligation of the thoracic duct is typically reserved when conservative measures and percutaneous embolization fails.

CARDIOPULMONARY COMPLICATIONS

A common cardiac complication in this patient population is atrial fibrillation (AF). Although AF may seem minor in comparison with some of the more grave acute complications, the literature indicates that this can be a marker of postoperative morbidity, including leaks, pulmonary complications, and mortality.[42] AF tends to occur in the immediate preoperative period and is associated with prolonged ICU stay and overall hospital length of stay.[43] It has even been associated with RLNP.[44]

Pneumonia and other pulmonary complications play a significant role in morbidity and mortality for the patient undergoing an esophagectomy. Postoperative pneumonia increases postoperative mortality by nearly 10% and decreases and diminishes 5-year overall survival by 12%.[44] Smokers seem to be at the greatest risk of developing pneumonia. Furthermore, baseline pulmonary dysfunction is a good predictor of postoperative pulmonary complications. Specifically, patients with a forced expiratory volume in 1 second less than 60% of predicted normal are greater than 3 times more likely to have a pulmonary complication after surgery.[45] Avoiding pulmonary complications can be difficult, because many patients undergoing esophagectomy have a history of smoking and, hence, diminished pulmonary reserve. Several studies have demonstrated that minimally invasive approaches improve pulmonary complications after esophagectomy.[46,47]

Prevention seems to be the key to pulmonary complications. Extrapolating from other thoracic operations, preoperative pulmonary optimization seems to decrease the risk of pneumonia and other pulmonary complications by half.[48,49] Aerobic exercise seems to have similar benefits.[50] Additional studies have demonstrated that poor functional status is associated with greater morbidity,[51,52] therefore it would seem that preoperative preparation greatly improves pulmonary outcomes for these complex cases. Other strategies include using thoracic epidurals and intraoperative protective ventilation approaches.[53]

LATE COMPLICATIONS
Anastomotic Strictures

Anastomotic strictures are not uncommon. They typically occur a few months after surgery but can present as soon as a few weeks. Presentation usually consist of significant dysphagia, persistent nausea, and difficulty with solid foods. Early strictures are usually related to ischemia at the anastomosis and can be treated with gentle endoscopic dilation. Later strictures are often associated with local tumor recurrence.[54] Strictures occurring more than 3 months after resection should be carefully evaluated by endoscopy for tumor recurrence. Dilation can provide short-lived relief, but these patients should be counseled that dysphagia will return.

Functional Dysphagia and Delayed Gastric Emptying

Functional dysphagia can also be classified as delayed gastric emptying. This can be due to a short remnant esophagus, muscle damage to the esophagus from surgical dissection, or nerve or vascular injury, which can cause a gastroparesis effect. Furthermore, accessory swallowing muscles can be injured during cervical dissection.[14] Denervation of the gastric conduit during mobilization can result in gastroparesis. Once performed with all gastric conduit mobilizations, routine pyloroplasty or pyloromyotomy is no longer performed by most esophageal surgeons. Persistent gastroparesis is commonly treated with endoscopic dilation or botulinum toxin infiltration into the pylorus. For patients with persistent gastroparesis that fails endoscopic management, surgical pyloroplasty should be considered.[55]

Reflux after Esophagectomy

When approaching the topic of reflux as a long-term complication after an esophagectomy, it is important to mention some of the risk factors. Ideally, a stomach conduit should be in the thorax; however, when the stomach is partially pulled with a significant portion remaining in the stomach, this may lead to increased incidence of reflux given the increase intraabdominal pressure. The nature of the procedure also lends itself to disrupting the natural reflux mechanism at the hiatus. Also exacerbating this problem is the presence of gastroparesis or delayed gastric emptying in this patient population.

Hiatal Hernias/Gastroesophageal Reflux

Patients who undergo gastric pull-up operations have a hiatal hernia (HH) by definition. Patients with symptomatic HH present with pain, dyspnea, vomiting, acute obstruction, dysphagia, or cough. The risk of HH after esophagectomy is 0.8% to 8%.[56,57] Although commonly performed, cruroplasty does not prevent formation of HH.[58] The most common location of HH is the left chest and may involve other intraabdominal organs, most commonly (but not limited to) the small and large bowel and the omentum. Some of these patients may require prompt intervention and resection for bowel ischemia in the case of strangulation. Minimally invasive approaches should be considered when repairing an HH, but the recurrence rate remains around 20%.[59]

Symptomatic HHs are more common after minimally invasive approaches.[56,60] This is believed to be a result of decreased adhesions with minimally invasive approaches, leading to greater organ mobility and potential for herniation, as well as increased intrathoracic pressure during laparoscopy artificially widening the esophageal hiatus.

Gastroesophageal reflux is common after esophagectomy.[61] Ideally, a gastric conduit should be in the thorax; however, when part of the stomach remains in the abdomen, increased abdominal pressure may lead to increased incidence of reflux.[62] The nature of the procedure also lends itself to disrupting the natural reflux mechanism at the hiatus. Also exacerbating this problem is the presence of gastroparesis or delayed gastric emptying in this patient population. Ant-acid medication along with diet modification is the mainstay in reflux therapy. Rarely should revisional surgery be considered.[63]

SUMMARY

It is clear that esophagectomies can be fraught with complications. Having knowledge about which complications to expect and their management can aid in minimizing their damaging, acute, and sometimes long-standing effects.

Acute complications such as anastomotic leaks, cardiopulmonary effects, and chyle leaks can lead to significant morbidity and mortality, and the threshold for suspicion and prompt intervention should remain low. There remain many unanswered questions in terms of specific pathophysiology for some of these complications. As surgeons continue to perfect their craft and decrease the morbidity and mortality associated with these procedures, continued efforts to analyze the associated complications must be made by remaining relentless in the search for an explanation in order to take a preventive approach when dealing with this patient population. Surgeons must understand that prevention begins at every aspect of the clinical phase, because scrupulous preoperative evaluation can prove to be lifesaving; however, this attention to detail should be carried through the intraoperative and postoperative phases. It is clear that minimally invasive approaches have provided significant benefit for patients and have aided in minimizing some acute complications; however, continued efforts must be made to find ways to manage and prevent those complications that are exacerbated by minimally invasive approaches. Evidence must continue to guide practice.

REFERENCES

1. Kamangar F, Dores GM, Anderson WF. Patterns of cancer incidence, mortality, and prevalence across five continents: defining priorities to reduce cancer disparities in different geographic regions of the world. J Clin Oncol 2006;24(14): 2137–50.
2. Jamieson GG, Mathew G, Ludemann R, et al. Postoperative mortality following oesophagectomy and problems in reporting its rate. Br J Surg 2004;91(8):943–7.
3. Low DE, Kuppusamy MK, Alderson D, et al. Benchmarking complications associated with esophagectomy. Ann Surg 2019;269(2):291–8.
4. Shen KR, Harrison-Phipps KM, Cassivi SD, et al. Esophagectomy after anti-reflux surgery. J Thorac Cardiovasc Surg 2010;139(4):969–75.
5. Bailey SH, Bull DA, Harpole DH, et al. Outcomes after esophagectomy: a ten-year prospective cohort. Ann Thorac Surg 2003;75(1):217–22 [discussion: 222].
6. Metzger R, Bollschweiler E, Vallbohmer D, et al. High volume centers for esophagectomy: what is the number needed to achieve low postoperative mortality? Dis Esophagus 2004;17(4):310–4.
7. Martin LW, Swisher SG, Hofstetter W, et al. Intrathoracic leaks following esophagectomy are no longer associated with increased mortality. Ann Surg 2005; 242(3):392–9 [discussion: 399–402].
8. Giuli R, Gignoux M. Treatment of carcinoma of the esophagus. Retrospective study of 2,400 patients. Ann Surg 1980;192(1):44–52.
9. Muller JM, Erasmi H, Stelzner M, et al. Surgical therapy of oesophageal carcinoma. Br J Surg 1990;77(8):845–57.
10. Sauvanet A, Baltar J, Le Mee J, et al. Diagnosis and conservative management of intrathoracic leakage after oesophagectomy. Br J Surg 1998;85(10):1446–9.
11. Whooley BP, Law S, Alexandrou A, et al. Critical appraisal of the significance of intrathoracic anastomotic leakage after esophagectomy for cancer. Am J Surg 2001;181(3):198–203.
12. Orringer MB, Marshall B, Iannettoni MD. Transhiatal esophagectomy: clinical experience and refinements. Ann Surg 1999;230(3):392–400 [discussion: 400–3].
13. Urschel JD. Esophagogastrostomy anastomotic leaks complicating esophagectomy: a review. Am J Surg 1995;169(6):634–40.
14. Chen KN. Managing complications I: leaks, strictures, emptying, reflux, chylothorax. J Thorac Dis 2014;6(Suppl 3):S355–63.
15. Patil PK, Patel SG, Mistry RC, et al. Cancer of the esophagus: esophagogastric anastomotic leak–a retrospective study of predisposing factors. J Surg Oncol 1992;49(3):163–7.
16. Doty JR, Salazar JD, Forastiere AA, et al. Postesophagectomy morbidity, mortality, and length of hospital stay after preoperative chemoradiation therapy. Ann Thorac Surg 2002;74(1):227–31 [discussion: 231].
17. Zacherl J, Sendler A, Stein HJ, et al. Current status of neoadjuvant therapy for adenocarcinoma of the distal esophagus. World J Surg 2003;27(9):1067–74.
18. Raman V, Moodie KL, Ofoche OO, et al. Endoscopy after esophagectomy: safety demonstrated in a porcine model. J Thorac Cardiovasc Surg 2017;154(3): 1152–8.

19. Aiko S, Yoshizumi Y, Sugiura Y, et al. Beneficial effects of immediate enteral nutrition after esophageal cancer surgery. Surg Today 2001;31(11):971–8.

20. Baigrie RJ, Devitt PG, Watkin DS. Enteral versus parenteral nutrition after oesophagogastric surgery: a prospective randomized comparison. Aust N Z J Surg 1996;66(10):668–70.

21. Mercer CD, Mungara A. Enteral feeding in esophageal surgery. Nutrition 1996; 12(3):200–1.

22. Weijs TJ, van Eden HWJ, Ruurda JP, et al. Routine jejunostomy tube feeding following esophagectomy. J Thorac Dis 2017;9(Suppl 8):S851–60.

23. Berkelmans GH, van Workum F, Weijs TJ, et al. The feeding route after esophagectomy: a review of literature. J Thorac Dis 2017;9(Suppl 8):S785–91.

24. Srinathan SK, Hamin T, Walter S, et al. Jejunostomy tube feeding in patients undergoing esophagectomy. Can J Surg 2013;56(6):409–14.

25. Bozzetti F, Braga M, Gianotti L, et al. Postoperative enteral versus parenteral nutrition in malnourished patients with gastrointestinal cancer: a randomised multicentre trial. Lancet 2001;358(9292):1487–92.

26. Braga M, Gianotti L, Vignali A, et al. Artificial nutrition after major abdominal surgery: impact of route of administration and composition of the diet. Crit Care Med 1998;26(1):24–30.

27. Peng J, Cai J, Niu ZX, et al. Early enteral nutrition compared with parenteral nutrition for esophageal cancer patients after esophagectomy: a meta-analysis. Dis Esophagus 2016;29(4):333–41.

28. Crestanello JA, Deschamps C, Cassivi SD, et al. Selective management of intrathoracic anastomotic leak after esophagectomy. J Thorac Cardiovasc Surg 2005; 129(2):254–60.

29. Paul S, Bueno R. Section VI: complications following esophagectomy: early detection, treatment, and prevention. Semin Thorac Cardiovasc Surg 2003; 15(2):210–5.

30. Dasari BV, Neely D, Kennedy A, et al. The role of esophageal stents in the management of esophageal anastomotic leaks and benign esophageal perforations. Ann Surg 2014;259(5):852–60.

31. Watkins JR, Farivar AS. Endoluminal therapies for esophageal perforations and leaks. Thorac Surg Clin 2018;28(4):541–54.

32. Dickinson KJ, Blackmon SH. Management of conduit necrosis following esophagectomy. Thorac Surg Clin 2015;25(4):461–70.

33. Lainas P, Fuks D, Gaujoux S, et al. Preoperative imaging and prediction of oesophageal conduit necrosis after oesophagectomy for cancer. Br J Surg 2017; 104(10):1346–54.

34. Sahebazamani M, Rubio E, Boyd M. Airway gastric fistula after esophagectomy for esophageal cancer. Ann Thorac Surg 2012;93(3):988–90.

35. Bartels HE, Stein HJ, Siewert JR. Tracheobronchial lesions following oesophagectomy: prevalence, predisposing factors and outcome. Br J Surg 1998; 85(3):403–6.

36. Scholtemeijer MG, Seesing MFJ, Brenkman HJF, et al. Recurrent laryngeal nerve injury after esophagectomy for esophageal cancer: incidence, management, and impact on short- and long-term outcomes. J Thorac Dis 2017;9(Suppl 8): S868–78.

37. Sachs PB, Zelch MG, Rice TW, et al. Diagnosis and localization of laceration of the thoracic duct: usefulness of lymphangiography and CT. AJR Am J Roentgenol 1991;157(4):703–5.

38. Bryant AS, Minnich DJ, Wei B, et al. The incidence and management of postoperative chylothorax after pulmonary resection and thoracic mediastinal lymph node dissection. Ann Thorac Surg 2014;98(1):232–5 [discussion: 235–7].

39. Orringer MB, Bluett M, Deeb GM. Aggressive treatment of chylothorax complicating transhiatal esophagectomy without thoracotomy. Surgery 1988;104(4): 720–6.

40. Majdalany BS, Khayat M, Downing T, et al. Lymphatic interventions for isolated, iatrogenic chylous ascites: a multi-institution experience. Eur J Radiol 2018; 109:41–7.

41. Kariya S, Nakatani M, Yoshida R, et al. Embolization for thoracic duct collateral leakage in high-output chylothorax after thoracic surgery. Cardiovasc Intervent Radiol 2017;40(1):55–60.

42. Stawicki SP, Prosciak MP, Gerlach AT, et al. Atrial fibrillation after esophagectomy: an indicator of postoperative morbidity. Gen Thorac Cardiovasc Surg 2011;59(6): 399–405.

43. Day RW, Jaroszewski D, Chang YH, et al. Incidence and impact of postoperative atrial fibrillation after minimally invasive esophagectomy. Dis Esophagus 2016; 29(6):583–8.

44. Booka E, Takeuchi H, Nishi T, et al. The impact of postoperative complications on survivals after esophagectomy for esophageal cancer. Medicine (Baltimore) 2015;94(33):e1369.

45. Shiozaki A, Fujiwara H, Okamura H, et al. Risk factors for postoperative respiratory complications following esophageal cancer resection. Oncol Lett 2012;3(4): 907–12.

46. Nozaki I, Mizusawa J, Kato K, et al. Impact of laparoscopy on the prevention of pulmonary complications after thoracoscopic esophagectomy using data from JCOG0502: a prospective multicenter study. Surg Endosc 2018;32(2): 651–9.

47. Nozaki I, Kato K, Igaki H, et al. Erratum to: evaluation of safety profile of thoracoscopic esophagectomy for T1bN0M0 cancer using data from JCOG0502: a prospective multicenter study. Surg Endosc 2015;29(12):3527.

48. Hulzebos EH, Helders PJ, Favie NJ, et al. Preoperative intensive inspiratory muscle training to prevent postoperative pulmonary complications in high-risk patients undergoing CABG surgery: a randomized clinical trial. JAMA 2006; 296(15):1851–7.

49. Katsura M, Kuriyama A, Takeshima T, et al. Preoperative inspiratory muscle training for postoperative pulmonary complications in adults undergoing cardiac and major abdominal surgery. Cochrane Database Syst Rev 2015;(10):CD010356.

50. Hulzebos EH, Smit Y, Helders PP, et al. Preoperative physical therapy for elective cardiac surgery patients. Cochrane Database Syst Rev 2012;(11):CD010118.

51. Baker S, Waldrop MG, Swords J, et al. Timed stair-climbing as a surrogate marker for sarcopenia measurements in predicting surgical outcomes. J Gastrointest Surg 2018. https://doi.org/10.1007/s11605-018-4042-0.

52. Reddy S, Contreras CM, Singletary B, et al. Timed stair climbing is the single strongest predictor of perioperative complications in patients undergoing abdominal surgery. J Am Coll Surg 2016;222(4):559–66.

53. Weijs TJ, Seesing MF, van Rossum PS, et al. Internal and external validation of a multivariable model to define hospital-acquired pneumonia after esophagectomy. J Gastrointest Surg 2016;20(4):680–7.

54. Sutcliffe RP, Forshaw MJ, Tandon R, et al. Anastomotic strictures and delayed gastric emptying after esophagectomy: incidence, risk factors and management. Dis Esophagus 2008;21(8):712–7.

55. Smith DS, Williams CS, Ferris CD. Diagnosis and treatment of chronic gastroparesis and chronic intestinal pseudo-obstruction. Gastroenterol Clin North Am 2003;32(2):619–58.

56. Price TN, Allen MS, Nichols FC 3rd, et al. Hiatal hernia after esophagectomy: analysis of 2,182 esophagectomies from a single institution. Ann Thorac Surg 2011;92(6):2041–5.

57. Kent MS, Luketich JD, Tsai W, et al. Revisional surgery after esophagectomy: an analysis of 43 patients. Ann Thorac Surg 2008;86(3):975–83 [discussion: 967–74].

58. Gooszen JAH, Slaman AE, van Dieren S, et al. Incidence and treatment of symptomatic diaphragmatic hernia after esophagectomy for cancer. Ann Thorac Surg 2018;106(1):199–206.

59. Ulloa Severino B, Fuks D, Christidis C, et al. Laparoscopic repair of hiatal hernia after minimally invasive esophagectomy. Surg Endosc 2016;30(3):1068–72.

60. Oor JE, Wiezer MJ, Hazebroek EJ. Hiatal hernia after open versus minimally invasive esophagectomy: a systematic review and meta-analysis. Ann Surg Oncol 2016;23(8):2690–8.

61. Kim D, Min YW, Park JG, et al. Influence of esophagectomy on the gastroesophageal reflux in patients with esophageal cancer. Dis Esophagus 2017;30(12):1–7.

62. Dai Z, He Q, Pan B, et al. Postoperative complication assessments of different reconstruction procedures after total pharyngolaryngoesophagectomy: tubular gastric pull-up versus whole gastric pull-up. Am Surg 2018;84(12):1927–31.

63. D'Journo XB, Martin J, Gaboury L, et al. Roux-en-Y diversion for intractable reflux after esophagectomy. Ann Thorac Surg 2008;86(5):1646–52.

Next-generation Sequencing in the Management of Gastric and Esophageal Cancers

Jill C. Rubinstein, MD, PhD, Norman G. Nicolson, MD,
Nita Ahuja, MD, MBA*

KEYWORDS

- Next-generation sequencing • Gastric and esophageal cancers
- High-throughput sequencing • Microsatellite instability

KEY POINTS

- Next-generation sequencing is changing the conception of gastric and esophageal malignancies, expanding the number of known genomic drivers and placing them in the context of oncogenic pathways.
- Currently, treatment of gastric adenocarcinoma differs from that of esophageal adenocarcinoma, but future genomically based classification schemes likely will supersede anatomic location in guiding management.
- The combination of genomic data with traditional clinical staging, including TNM and histopathologic variables, has the potential to inform more effective, individualized treatment plans.

INTRODUCTION

Cancer is a disease of the genome, arising out of a sophisticated interplay between thousands of genes, forming intricate pathways to carry out all levels of cellular function and subject to the lifelong influence of varied and unpredictable environmental factors. There are myriad routes of oncogenesis, reflecting complex interactions between forces acting at the level of the DNA sequence and its epigenetic framework, the gene expression machinery and subsequent RNA processing, and the protein itself. There is the power to interrogate all of these processes on a genome-wide scale using high-throughput technologies, such as next-generation sequencing (NGS). The number of raw data points generated through these experiments, coupled with the necessity of integrating multiple levels of data to discern meaningful information, brings

Disclosure: Dr. Ahuja has received grant funding from Cepheid and Astex and has served as consultant to Ethicon. She has licensed methylation biomarkers to Cepheid.
Department of Surgery, Yale University, School of Medicine, PO Box 208062, New Haven, CT 06520, USA
* Corresponding author.
E-mail address: nita.ahuja@yale.edu

about a combinatorial explosion of analytical dimensions. The sheer size of these data sets is a humbling illustration of the magnitude of the task: to identify recurrent patterns amid the sea of available data and to exploit them for clinical gain.

Malignancy of the foregut is common and carries a poor prognosis, with overall 5-year survival rates of 18.8% and 30.6% in the esophagus and stomach, respectively.[1] Management paradigms vary dramatically between primary esophageal tumors and gastric tumors, and few targeted therapies exist for either. With increasing knowledge of the genomic underpinnings of upper gastrointestinal malignancies, driven largely by the utilization of high-throughput sequencing technologies, more sophisticated, molecularly based classification systems are being developed, in the hope of devising rational treatment approaches based more on a tumor's specific genomic drivers than on its anatomic site.

A SURGEON'S GUIDE TO THE VOCABULARY OF GENOMICS

Every cell carries within it its own genome the collection of DNA that encodes every protein produced by the organism. DNA is made up of long chains of paired nucleotides, wrapped into the signature double helix, and further folded and wrapped around specialized proteins called histones. Human DNA is carried on 23 pairs of chromosomes (as well as a small complement of mitochondrial DNA) and stored in the cell's nucleus. The human genome consists of approximately 3 billion DNA base pairs, approximately 1% to 2% of which encode proteins. DNA is transcribed into RNA, which is then translated into proteins.

A majority of genetic diseases are due to alterations in the protein-coding portion of the genome, known as the *exome*. Genomic alterations include single-nucleotide variations, which may be synonymous (meaning the encoded amino acid is unchanged) or nonsynonymous (meaning a change in the produced protein) (**Table 1**). Short insertions or deletions (indels) in the DNA sequence may result in shifts in translation reading frame (often producing a truncated or nonfunctional protein) or an insertion or deletion of 1 or more amino acids, with varying effect. Single-nucleotide variations or indels, which are noted within the spectrum of normal human variation, are often referred to as single-nucleotide polymorphisms, and are an important source of understanding in population-level genetics. Mutations may be carried in a patient's germline, meaning inherited from parental DNA and carried by every cell throughout the organism, or somatic, meaning specific to a particular cell or tissue, such as a cancer-defining mutation carried by tumor cells but not neighboring normal cells.

Beyond single-nucleotide polymorphisms, entire regions of the genome may be deleted or duplicated (or tripled, quadrupled, and so forth), resulting in copy number alterations, which may have varying effects on protein production. If 1 allele is deleted and the other duplicated, the locus is said to have suffered loss of heterozygosity, which is particularly important if the normal allele is lost while a mutant allele is doubled. Genes may be cut off from their typical position and stuck into another place in the genome, resulting in a fusion gene product. Finally, a mutation in a gene involved in DNA repair may be the beginning of a chain reaction, causing innumerable additional mutations as because cells are unable to successfully repair routine DNA replication errors.

One such class of mutations results in the so-called microsatellite instability (MSI), seen across a variety of human cancers, in which repetitive, usually noncoding DNA regions, called *microsatellites* (particularly vulnerable to DNA repair errors), change in length due to slippage of DNA polymerases during DNA replication. With the rise of cancer immunotherapy, it has become increasingly clear that although

Table 1
Essential next-generation sequencing terms

Next-generation sequencing techniques	
WES	Provides single-nucleotide resolution across protein-coding regions of genome
Whole-genome sequencing	Similar to exome sequencing but covers all bases in the genome
Targeted sequencing	Similar to exome sequencing but targets a limited subset of candidate genes
Gene expression profiling	Relative level of RNA for each gene; may have more functional association but possibly influenced by cell environment
RNA sequencing	Similar to gene expression analysis, but also includes sequence data of each RNA transcript
Types of genetic alterations	
Single-nucleotide variation	Single base change, such as from C to T or G to A
Indel	Short insertion or deletion of several base pairs; may result in frameshift or insertion/deletion of amino acids
Copy number alteration	Deletion or amplification of a region of the genome
Loss of heterozygosity	Deletion of 1 allele and amplification of the other allele for a given gene
Gene fusion	Breakage and recombination of separate DNA sequences, resulting in chimeric fusion transcript
MSI	Consequence of failure of DNA repair, resulting in inability to repair routine DNA replication errors and extensive changes in repetitive DNA regions (microsatellites)

hypermutated tumors (including MSI and other non-MSI hypermutators) may be more intrinsically aggressive owing to high numbers of potential driving mutations, the resulting mutated proteins, when expressed at the cell surface, function as neoantigens, driving an antitumor immune response as immune cells identify these proteins as nonself. This natural immune response can be augmented with checkpoint inhibitors, such as pembrolizumab.[2]

In addition to these sources of genetic variation, each cell adjusts to its environment through epigenetic modifications, which modify gene expression without being directly encoded in the DNA sequence. For example, some bases can be methylated, which can alter expression of neighboring genes. Other genes are regulated by modification of DNA structure and associated proteins, such as histones, which allow DNA to be available for transcription (euchromatin) or tightly bound for storage (heterochromatin), depending on the identity and needs of the cell. Epigenetics are responsible for the tremendous diversity in cell structure and function seen throughout a given organism despite the shared and largely invariant genetic code.

A PRIMER ON NEXT-GENERATION SEQUENCING

First-generation sequencing technology, also known as Sanger sequencing, refers to the selective incorporation of chain-terminating dideoxynucleotides during in vitro replication of a single-stranded DNA template to discern its sequence.[3] In batch mode, automated Sanger sequencing instruments can sequence a few hundred samples at a time. In contrast, second-generation sequencing (NGS) uses high-throughput methods that produce millions to billions of reads per run.[4] A major advantage of these methods in cancer genomics is the ability to study the entire genome simultaneously, eliminating the bias of interrogating only selected cancer genes and opening the potential to discover novel targets. There are 3 widely used commercial platforms for NGS, including Solexa (Illumina, San Diego, CA), 454 Genome Sequencer (Roche Applied Science, Penzberg, Germany), and the SOLiD platform (ThermoFisher, Waltham, MA). Regardless of the platform used, the basic principle underlying NGS is that of massively parallel, cyclic interrogation of short, clonally expanded DNA sequences that are fixed in space.[5] The basic steps of NGS are as follows[4,6]:

- Library preparation: random fragmentation of DNA, ligation of common adaptor sequences
- Cluster generation: polymerase chain reaction amplification of each library component on a spatially fixed array
- Sequencing: massively parallel, enzyme-driven biochemical and imaging-based data processing
- Data analysis: alignment of short reads to reference genome, variant detection

Although sequencing of the whole genome is technically feasible and is becoming increasingly common in the research setting, *whole-exome sequencing* (*WES*) and targeted sequencing are more routinely encountered in clinical practice. These techniques target the exome (all protein-coding regions of the genome) or a prespecified set of cancer-associated genes and take advantage of high-throughput methods at a fraction of the cost and computational requirements of whole-genome sequencing (**Fig. 1**). Technology that is affordable and that rapidly produces billions of short sequence reads presents several logistical challenges for the processing and storage of data. Beyond these considerations, there are inherent pitfalls when analyzing large data; the "curse of dimensionality" refers to the observation that as the number of variables being studied increases, the amount of data required to draw statistically sounds conclusions increases exponentially.[7] For cancer genomics studies, this means there is an inherent imbalance between the ability to generate vast molecular data sets and the small number of patients available for analysis. This phenomenon in no way precludes the meaningful study of cancer genomics through massively parallel techniques but rather demands new paradigms of analysis and a multidisciplinary approach, including researchers with expertise in handling high-dimensional data. Increasingly, such investigations are moving out of the laboratory and into the clinic, such that there is a need not only for surgeon-scientists to drive the generation of new genomics-derived knowledge but also for practicing surgical oncologists to begin to understand these methodologies as the information becomes available and actionable for patients. Several genetic alterations have been described in gastric and esophageal cancers, and there is a race to determine which of these are actionable mutations for therapeutic efficacy (**Table 2**).[8,9]

HISTOPATHOLOGIC CLASSIFICATION OF GASTRIC ADENOCARCINOMA

Traditionally, classification of gastric adenocarcinoma (AC) is by histopathology, using the Lauren[10] criteria to distinguish 2 major subtypes: intestinal and diffuse. The intestinal type is generally associated with *Helicobacter pylori* infection and arises from chronic gastritis and intestinal metaplasia, whereas the diffuse type shows widely distributed cells, sometimes signet ring, with submucosal infiltration. The World Health Organization classification system is also based on classical histopathology and includes 4 subcategories: tubular, papillary, mucinous, and poorly cohesive/signet ring.[11] These classification schemata have some clinical utility in their ability to predict

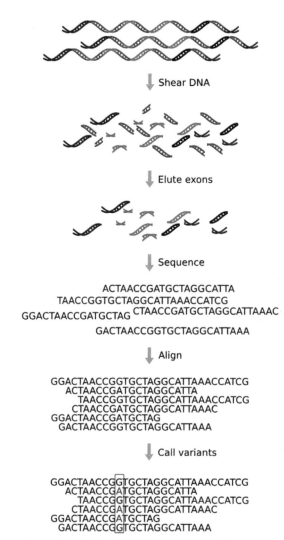

Fig. 1. Simplified schematic of WES, the most common NGS approach. Genomic DNA is sheared, exons are collected and sequenced, and reads are aligned to the reference genome, allowing for variant calling. Variants are further filtered to highlight those most likely to have functional consequences for the cell, depending on the research or clinical setting in question.

tumor behavior, but there currently are no specific management paradigms based specifically on this subtyping. It has long been understood that a small subset of diffuse/signet ring cell tumors are familial, resulting from germline mutation in E-cadherin (*CDH1*). Testing for mutation in this gene was among the first genetically informed clinical practices in gastric cancer, and, although it is altered in only a small minority of patients, all practitioners treating this disease should be familiar with indications for *CDH1* screening (**Table 3**).[12,13]

Molecular classification of gastric tumors using NGS technology provides a powerful adjunct to traditional histopathologic classification. These technologies hold

Table 2
Common genetic alterations in gastroesophageal adenocarcinomas and esophageal squamous cell carcinomas

Gastroesophageal Adenocarcinoma		Esophageal Squamous Carcinoma	
Gene	Alteration Frequency (%)	Gene	Alteration Frequency (%)
TP53	14–59	TP53	60–93
PIK3CA	7–36	CCND1	33–46
CDH1	4–36	CDKN2A	12–47
ERBB2 (HER2)	2–32	KRAS	5–27
ARID1A	8–27	FAT1	14–27
PTEN	0–27	KMT2D	19–26
KRAS	0–27	EGFR	6–24
RHOA	0–23	TERT	0–22
APC	3–14	NOTCH1	9–19
ERBB3	0–10	RB1	0–11
CTNNB1	2–9	PIK3CA	4–10
MET	0–9	MYC	0–9
FBXW7	2–6		
SMAD4	4–6		
EGFR	0–6		
NRAS	0–5		
MSI[a]	22–23		

[a] MSI is not a specific gene but a pattern of DNA alterations, often associated with mutations in DNA repair genes.

Data from Harada K, Mizrak Kaya D, Shimodaira Y, et al. Translating genomic profiling to gastrointestinal cancer treatment. Future Oncol 2017;13(10):919–34; and Lee HS, Kim WH, Kwak Y, et al. Molecular testing for gastrointestinal cancer. J Pathol Transl Med 2017;51(2):103–21.

promise for the discovery of biomarkers that may predict tumor behavior, response to therapy, or likelihood of recurrence. Additionally, expanding the scope and resolution with which the tumor genome is investigated promises to identify new molecular targets for therapy.

Table 3
International Gastric Cancer Linkage Consortium guidelines for familial germline *CDH1* testing

Family[a] *CDH1* screening recommended	• At least 2 cases in the family of gastric cancer at any age, if at least 1 is diffuse • A single case of diffuse gastric cancer prior to age 40 • Personal or family history of diffuse gastric cancer and lobular breast cancer, with at least 1 prior to age 50
Consider family[a] *CDH1* screening	• Bilateral lobular breast cancer or family history of 2 or more cases of lobular breast cancer prior to age 50 • Personal or family history of diffuse gastric cancer and cleft lip/palate in the same patient • In situ signet ring histology or pagetoid spread of signet ring cells

[a] Including first-degree or second-degree relatives.

MOLECULAR CLASSIFICATION OF GASTRIC ADENOCARCINOMA

The first exome sequencing study in gastric cancer was published in 2011 and included 22 patients.[14] Despite a limited cohort size, the study identified a list of 20 candidate genes, including the previously known drivers *TP53*, *PTEN*, and *CTNNB1*. In addition, the chromatin remodeling family gene *ARID1A* was significantly enriched for inactivating mutations. Analysis for the most perturbed gene pathways also identified those involved in chromatin modification as commonly mutated. A subsequent study used functional knock-down assays to confirm the role of *ARID1A* in suppressing cell proliferation, providing strong support for its role as a candidate tumor suppressor gene in gastric cancer.[15]

COMPREHENSIVE PROFILING DEFINES MOLECULAR CATEGORIES OF GASTRIC CANCER

The Cancer Genome Atlas (TCGA) Research Network proposed a genomic classification system for gastric cancer based on analysis of 295 samples. This is the most comprehensive study to date, using multiple high-throughput technologies, including DNA sequencing and copy number analysis, messenger RNA and microRNA sequencing, and a protein-level assay.[16] The proposed system includes 4 distinct subtypes; tumors that are Epstein-Barr virus positive (EBV+) are distinguished from those that demonstrate MSI, genomic stability (GS), and chromosomal instability (CIN) **(Fig. 2, Table 4)**. Although there was no observed difference in overall survival between the subgroups, the classification correlates with specific clinical characteristics, including tumor location, age, and gender. Additionally, the study suggests several alternative pathways for gastric tumorigenesis, thus serving as a hypothesis generator, suggesting potential future therapeutic targets for appropriately selected patients.

GENE EXPRESSION–BASED CLASSIFICATION SYSTEM FOR GASTRIC CANCER

An alternative classification system was devised by the Asian Cancer Research Group (ACRG) using gene expression profiling from a cohort of 300 primary gastric cancer

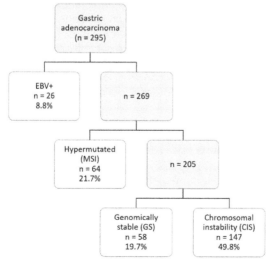

Fig. 2. TCGA molecular classification system. Using comprehensive molecular profiling, gastric tumors are divided into 4 categories based on the presence of EBV infection, MSI, and GS.

Table 4
The Cancer Genome Atlas molecular classification of gastric cancer with salient features of each subtype

The Cancer Genome Atlas Classification	Defining Characteristics
EBV+	• *PIK3CA, ARID1A, TP53* mutation • *PD-L1/L2* overexpression • CpG island methylator phenotype • *CDKN2A* silencing • Increased immune cell signaling • More frequently in fundus and body • Male predominance
MSI	• Hypermutation • *TP53, KRAS, PIK3A, ARID1A* mutation • CpG island methylator phenotype • *MLH1* silencing • Mitotic pathways • Diagnosed at older age • Female predominance
GS	• Diffuse histology • *CDH1, RHOA* mutations • CLDN18-ARHGAP fusion • Increased expression of cell adhesion pathways • Diagnosed at earlier age
CIN	• Intestinal histology • Aneuploidy • *TP53* mutation • RTK-RAS activation • More frequently at Gastroesophageal-junction and cardia

samples.[17,18] Four distinct subtypes were identified based on the presence or absence of MSI, epithelial-to-mesenchymal transition (EMT), and TP53 activity (**Fig. 3, Table 5**). These subtypes demonstrated significant associations with multiple clinical factors, including age, tumor location, grade, and American Joint Committee on Cancer stage. In addition, correlations could be made with the traditional Lauren classification systems: MSS/EMT tumors were primarily of the diffuse subtype, whereas a large fraction of the MSI tumors were intestinal. The relationship between this expression-based molecular classification system and the Lauren system illustrates the power of high-throughput technology to help bridge the gap between genotype and phenotype, identifying potential genomic phenomena that are driving histopathologic characteristics.

In contrast to the TCGA-derived classifications, the ACRG-defined subtypes were significantly associated with overall survival, a trend that was validated using 3 independent gastric cancer cohorts.[16,19,20] The best survival was noted in the MSI group, followed by MSS/TP53+ subsets, MSS/TP53− subsets, and finally the MSS/EMT subset ($P<.0004$ by univariate log-rank test), and the influence of molecular subtype on survival was robust ($P<.02$), even when accounting for stage, histology, and other traditional clinical factors in multivariable analysis. Yet, the challenge remains in deriving clinically useful information from these molecular classification systems, in particular those based on multidimensional mutation and expression profiles, which may be too costly and time consuming to be of clinical utility.

It is important to keep focus on the strength of these large-scale investigations, which is their ability to identify patterns in multidimensional data that otherwise are

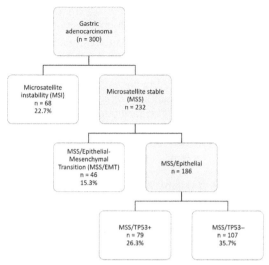

Fig. 3. ACRG molecular classification system. Using gene expression profiling, gastric tumors are divided into 4 categories based on the presence of MSI, EMT, and TP53 activity.

outside the capacity of the human brain to discern. The described classification schemes represent a distillation of millions of data points into simple categories, providing a more accessible framework to approach the complexity that underscores cancer genomics. In this sense, NGS technologies can be thought of as tools for the generation of hypotheses, identifying potential targets for downstream study and eventually clinical intervention.

DATA POOLING PROVIDES DEEPER INSIGHT INTO GASTRIC CANCER GENOMICS

As discussed previously, there is an inherent problem of dimensionality in dealing with NGS data. The number of data points studied is orders of magnitude greater

Table 5
Asian Cancer Research Group molecular classification of gastric cancer with salient features of each subtype

Asian Cancer Research Group Classification	Defining Characteristics
MSI	• Heavy mutational burden • Predominantly in antrum • Primarily intestinal histology • Best overall survival, earliest stage at diagnosis • Higher rate of liver-limited recurrence
MSS/EMT	• Lowest mutational burden • Younger age • Primarily diffuse histology • Worst overall survival, higher stage at diagnosis • Highest rate of recurrence, peritoneal spread
MSS/TP53+	• Highest percentage EBV+ tumors • Second-best overall survival
MSS/TP53−	• Higher rate of liver-limited recurrence

than the number of available samples, with the resultant dilemma that multiple hypothesis testing at such a high dimension will identify seemingly improbable events purely by chance. Even with rigorous statistical analysis, it has been estimated that between 600 and 5000 samples of a given tumor type, depending on the background mutation frequency, are required to reliably identify recurrently mutated genes.[21] The genomics community has recognized the necessity of combining cohorts to achieve adequately powered analyses, responding with the development of sophisticated platforms for genomic data pooling that facilitate data aggregation and processing through common bioinformatics pipelines. The Genomic Data Commons, hosted by the National Cancer Institute, is 1 such data repository, providing unified access and Web-based analytical tools to improve the accessibility of these Goliath data sets.[22]

Demonstrating the power of combining data sets, Li and colleagues[23] integrated mutational profiles and clinicopathologic data from multiple recent sequencing studies to produce a cohort of 544 gastric cancer samples.[14,18,24,25] Tumors were classified as either hypermutated (13.2%) or regular-mutated (86.8%), with significant enrichment for samples with MSI in the former group. The regular group was further subdivided into 2 subsets based on patterns of significantly mutated genes. The first regular group was enriched for multiple previously implicated cancer genes, including *TP53*, *XIRP2*, and *APC*, and was associated with significantly better survival; the second subgroup was overrepresented by alterations in *ARID1A*, *CDH1*, *PIK3CA*, *ERBB2*, and *RHOA*. The integrated molecular data set also provided greater statistical power to discover genes mutated at lower frequency that were previously unrecognized as significantly mutated in gastric cancer (eg, *FBXW7*, *XIRP2*, *NBEA*, *COL14A1*, *CNBD1*, *AKAP6*, and *ITGAV*). Finally, the combined cohort confirms the significance of *CDH1* as a poor prognostic marker in diffuse-type gastric cancer but not in intestinal-type gastric cancer. The confirmation of this known driver demonstrates that, in addition to investigating large-scale patterns in the data, adequately powered high-throughput studies are able to identify individual candidate genes for further downstream study.

HISTOPATHOLOGIC CLASSIFICATION OF ESOPHAGEAL CANCER

A majority of esophageal malignancies are either squamous cell carcinoma (SCC) or AC, 2 categories that are associated with distinct anatomic sites, environmental risk factors, natural history, and treatment outcomes.[26] Esophageal SCC originates predominantly in the upper two-thirds of the esophagus, and risk is increased by chronic exposure to tobacco and alcohol. In contrast, esophageal AC tends to arise in the distal esophagus, near the gastroesophageal junction (GEJ) and is associated with chronic acid reflux and Barrett esophagus.[27] Histopathologically, SCC develops from progression of epithelial dysplasia to carcinoma in situ and ultimately invasive disease,[28] whereas AC arises in the context of intestinal metaplasia and parallels the growth pattern seen in Lauren intestinal-type gastric AC.[29] The distinct behaviors of these 2 main categories of disease has led to controversy over whether SCC and AC of the esophagus should be conceived of as separate entities, both for the purpose of research and in clinical management.[27,30]

MOLECULAR CHARACTERIZATION OF ESOPHAGEAL SQUAMOUS CELL CARCINOMA

Several current mutations have been implicated in esophageal SCC, including those causing loss of function of the tumor suppressor genes *TP53* and *NOTCH1* and activating mutations in the AKT signaling pathway gene *PIK3CA*.[31,32] A 2014 study of 139 esophageal SCC patients, using high-throughput technologies, confirmed these previously identified genes and discovered a group of previously unknown mutated genes, including *FAT1*, *FAT2*, *ZNF750*, and *KMT2D*.[33] The FAT family of proteins belong to the cadherin superfamily, which are involved in both cell-cell adhesion and cell-cell signaling. *KMT2D* is in the histone methyltransferase family, which functions in chromatin remodeling. *ZNF750* is a transcription factor involved in epithelial differentiation in the TP63 pathway. Both the histone methyltransferase and FAT cadherin families are known to harbor somatic mutations in several cancer types.[34,35]

MOLECULAR CHARACTERIZATION OF ESOPHAGEAL ADENOCARCINOMA

Numerous somatic mutations have been reported in esophageal AC, including some of the same candidates noted in the SCC group, such as the tumor suppressor *TP53* and the oncogene *PIK3CA*.[36,37] In a 2013 WES study of 149 esophageal AC samples, Dulak and colleagues[38] confirmed the presence these *TP53* and *PIK3CA* variants as well as other previously identified candidate genes *CDKN2A*, *SMAD4*, and *ARID1A*. *PIK3CA* was the most frequently mutated gene among the subset for which therapeutic inhibitors have either been approved for clinical use or are in development. Loss of function mutations of chromatin-remodeling genes also were commonly noted (*SPG20*, *TLR4*, *ELMO1*, and *DOCK2*), with functional downstream assays confirming the potential for increased invasion and motility associated with *ELMO1* and *DOCK2* mutation.

GENOMIC DISTINCTIONS BETWEEN ESOPHAGEAL SQUAMOUS CELL CARCINOMA AND ADENOCARCINOMA

This recent attention to high-throughput interrogation of esophageal cancer genomes provides further insight into the genomic differences between SCC and AC and may become more informative for treatment planning than traditional anatomic and histopathologic considerations. In a 2017 study, TCGA Research Group performed a comprehensive molecular analysis of 164 esophageal carcinomas, including both SCC and AC.[39] They noted that the molecular features of esophageal SCC more closely resembled that of head and neck SCC than esophageal AC (**Fig. 4**). The SCCs demonstrated up-regulation of the Wnt, syndecan, and p63 pathways, in contrast to increased signaling in CDH1 and related regulatory pathways (ARF6 and FOXA) in the ACs. Notably, *ERBB2* was altered in 32% of ACs compared with only 3% of SCCs. Silencing of *CDKN2A* was a common event, having an impact on 76% of both tumor types, but the mechanism varied; a majority of SCCs were silenced via deletion, whereas in AC activity was lost due to a combination of epigenetic silencing, deletion, and missense mutation.

To explore the genomic relationship between ACs of different anatomic location, the TCGA study also included 359 gastric ACs and 36 tumors, which spanned the GEJ. The molecular profile of esophageal AC was found similar to that of the chromosomally unstable variant of gastric AC (CIN subtype), highlighting a blurred genomic boundary between the 2 entities. Epigenetic analysis did demonstrate an increasing propensity for hypermethylation in the esophageal tumors and more proximal GEJ tumors, including a higher incidence of *CDKN2A* silencing. Overall, the findings from this comprehensive analysis suggest that esophageal cancers and CIN gastric cancers should be conceived of as highly similar entities. In contrast, esophageal SCC and esophageal AC are more appropriately treated as 2 separate diseases and should not be considered together for the purpose of clinical trials.

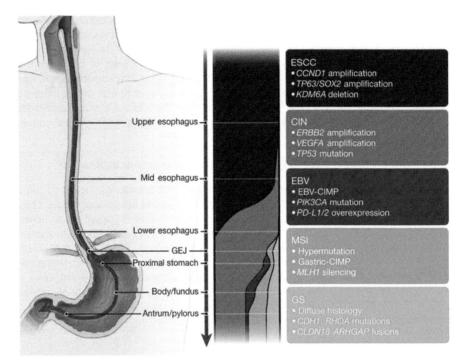

Fig. 4. Anatomic correlate of genomic subtypes of gastroesophageal carcinomas. CIMP, CpG island methylator phenotype; ESCC, esophageal squamous cell carcinoma. (*From* Cancer Genome Atlas Research Network; Analysis Working Group: Asan University, BC Cancer Agency, et al. Integrated genomic characterization of oesophageal carcinoma. Nature 2017;541(7636):174; with permission.)

TARGETED THERAPY IN GASTRIC AND ESOPHAGEAL CANCERS

Comparative analysis of the molecular signatures of gastric and esophageal cancers has also identified patterns implicating numerous potential oncogenic drivers. This high-resolution genomic characterization complements traditional histopathologic classifiers and provides a basis to explore rational treatment planning based on known targets. Importantly, even for tumor types that share common oncogenic pathways, the nature of the perturbation often varies, which may suggest the need for therapeutic approaches that are tailored to the specific functional mechanism of genomic alteration. For example, chromatin-modifying enzymes were a common target in both esophageal SCC and esophageal AC, but the specific affected genes varied by tumor type. Additionally, *CDKN2A* silencing occurred through deletion in SCC but through multiple mechanisms in AC, mainly epigenetic silencing.[39]

Among the earliest developments in the individualized treatment of gastric AC and esophageal AC was specific targeting of tumors with *HER-2* overexpression. Through heterodimerization with other ErbB family receptors, HER-2 activates *RAS-MAPK* and *PI3K-ALT* pathways. The rate of HER-2 amplification reported in these tumors varies widely in the literature, with a mean reported incidence of 17.9% (range 4.4%–53.4%).[40] A 2010 phase 3, randomized controlled trial Trastuzumab for Gastric Cancer (ToGA) demonstrated improved median survival with trastuzumab in combination with chemotherapy compared with chemotherapy alone (13.8 months vs 11.1 months) for metastatic gastric or GEJ tumors with HER2 overexpression[41,42]; however, the treatment response was not durable on updated survival analysis (**Fig. 5**).[42] These early data led to several additional trials that are currently under way (for summary, see Young and Chau[43] and Kankeu Fonkoua and Yee[42]). With this increasing number of trials, it is essential that providers make testing for *HER-2* amplification as much a part of providers standard care in foregut malignancy as it is in breast cancer.

Another targeted therapy came in the form of the monoclonal antibody ramucirumab, which is an antagonist of the vascular endothelial growth factor signaling pathway. The REGARD trial was a phase 3, randomized controlled trial that demonstrated improved overall survival (median 5.2 months vs 3.8 months) in advanced gastric cancer patients who progressed after first-line chemotherapy.[44] In the RAINBOW trial, ramucirumab in combination with paclitaxel also demonstrated improved median overall survival over paclitaxel alone (9.6 months vs 7.4 months).[45] Bevacizumab is another monoclonal antibody to vascular endothelial growth factor, showing encouraging early results in gastric AC and GEJ AC[46]; however, esophageal SCC has not been studied extensively due to the severe toxicity demonstrated in trials of SCC of the lung, specifically life-threatening hemoptysis.[47]

One promising avenue for targeted therapy is in the emerging area of immunotherapy. Programmed cell death protein 1 (PD-1) is a receptor expressed mainly on activated T cells that binds to its ligands (PD-L1 and PD-L2) and down-regulates the immune response, including suppression of antitumor immunity. As discussed previously, it is hypothesized that tumors with high mutational burden due to mismatch repair defects or MSI have increased potential to express nonself antigens

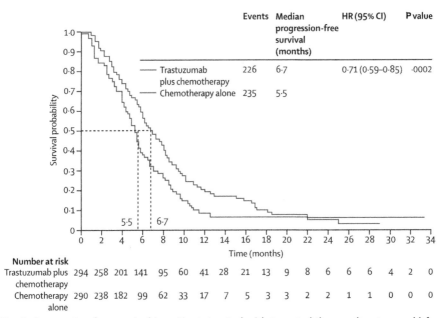

Fig. 5. Progression-free survival in patients treated with targeted therapy (trastuzumab) for metastatic gastric cancer. HR, hazard ratio. (*From* Bang YJ, Van Cutsem E, Feyereislova A, et al. Trastuzumab in combination with chemotherapy versus chemotherapy alone for treatment of HER2-positive advanced gastric or gastro-oesophageal junction cancer (ToGA): a phase 3, open-label, randomised controlled trial. Reprinted with permission from Elsevier [Lancet 2010;376(9742):690].)

and would be susceptible to immune checkpoint blockade.[2] A 2017 study based on this premise tested the efficacy of the anti–PD-1 monoclonal antibody, pembrolizumab, in mismatch repair–deficient versus mismatch repair–proficient tumors, mainly colorectal. The study showed that mismatch repair deficiency was associated with a response to immune checkpoint blockade, and a follow-up study using 12 different tumor types demonstrated that this finding was independent of the tissue of origin.[2,48] The phase 1b KEYNOTE-012 trial tested pembrolizumab in PD-L1–positive recurrent or metastatic gastric ACs and GEJ ACs.[49] The toxicity profile was deemed manageable and antitumor activity promising enough that further phase 2 and phase 3 trials are under way. Immune checkpoint inhibition in the form of anti–CTLA-4 monoclonal antibodies has also been investigated in gastric and GEJ cancers but with limited numbers and disappointing results to date.[50]

These targeted therapies represent modest advances at best, with only a minority of patients achieving a response, but newer classification schemes, generated through high-throughput molecular studies, such as those reviewed in this article, may suggest subtypes of tumors that are most likely to derive benefit. For example, the EBV+ gastric subtype defined in the TCGA study demonstrated high levels of PD-L1/L2 expression, indicating that this population might be best suited for targeted therapy with anti–PD-1 monoclonal antibodies.[16] Further candidate gene targets specific to each TCGA-defined and ACRG-defined subtype are tabulated by Kankeu Fonkoua and Yee,[42] demonstrating distinct but overlapping lists of targeted agents.

SUMMARY

In recent decades, there has been a shift in the predominant anatomic location of both esophageal cancers and gastric cancers, resulting in a greater percentage of lower esophageal ACs and proximal gastric ACs. This evolution in tumor location and histology suggests that esophageal AC and gastric AC might more accurately be grouped together, with esophageal SCC considered a separate disease entity. New classification systems based on molecular subcategorization derived from high-throughput sequencing technologies provides strong support for this notion.

As knowledge of the molecular pathways underlying gastric and esophageal cancers continues to grow, the pressure increases to find effective ways to translate this understanding into clinically meaningful advances. With the addition of NGS technology, several known tumor drivers have been confirmed and numerous additional candidate genes have been identified. The ability to assess the entire genome simultaneously also allows these individual genomic insults to be contextualized within the pathways to which they contribute, opening avenues for additional potential therapeutic targets. Improved molecular classification of tumors and further biomarker discovery have the potential to guide more personalized management decisions, but many challenges remain in translating this new insight regarding the molecular underpinnings of these groups of tumors into clinically meaningful advances. Although clinical practice patterns may be slow to change, the reality is that patients' tumors are increasingly undergoing sequencing analysis in the clinical setting. Surgeons have grown comfortable incorporating gene mutation data from single genes, or small panels of genes, into management algorithms. With ever-growing panels of genes being interrogated, it is incumbent on surgeons as a community to gain sufficient fluency in the basics of high-throughput technologies so that practice paradigms keep pace with the current state of cancer genomics, and patients reap the potential benefits of these advances.

REFERENCES

1. Howlader N, Noone AM, Krapcho M, et al. SEER cancer statistics review, 1975-2014, National Cancer Institute. Bethesda (MD): National Cancer Institute; 2017.
2. Le DT, Uram JN, Wang H, et al. PD-1 blockade in tumors with mismatch-repair deficiency. N Engl J Med 2015;372(26):2509–20.
3. Sanger F, Coulson AR. A rapid method for determining sequences in DNA by primed synthesis with DNA polymerase. J Mol Biol 1975;94(3):441–8.
4. Goodwin S, McPherson JD, McCombie WR. Coming of age: ten years of next-generation sequencing technologies. Nat Rev Genet 2016;17(6):333–51.
5. Castiblanco J. A primer on current and common sequencing technologies. In: Anaya J, Shoenfeld Y, Rojas-Villarraga A, editors. Autoimmunity: from bench to bedside. Bogota (Colombia): El Rosario University Press; 2013. Chapter 47.
6. Rusk N, Kiermer V. Primer: sequencing–the next generation. Nat Methods 2008; 5(1):15.
7. Bellman RE. Dynamic programming. Princeton (NJ): Princeton University Press; 1957.
8. Harada K, Mizrak Kaya D, Shimodaira Y, et al. Translating genomic profiling to gastrointestinal cancer treatment. Future Oncol 2017;13(10):919–34.
9. Lee HS, Kim WH, Kwak Y, et al. Molecular testing for gastrointestinal cancer. J Pathol Transl Med 2017;51(2):103–21.
10. Lauren P. The two histological main types of gastric carcinoma: diffuse and so-called intestinal-type carcinoma. an attempt at a histo-clinical classification. Acta Pathol Microbiol Scand 1965;64:31–49.
11. Aaltonen LA, Hamilton SR. Pathology and genetics of tumours of the digestive system. In: Redo U, Underline BI, Superscript S, et al, editors. World Health Organization classification of tumours. Lyon (France): IARC Press; 2000.
12. Brooks-Wilson AR, Kaurah P, Suriano G, et al. Germline E-cadherin mutations in hereditary diffuse gastric cancer: assessment of 42 new families and review of genetic screening criteria. J Med Genet 2004;41(7):508–17.
13. van der Post RS, Vogelaar IP, Carneiro F, et al. Hereditary diffuse gastric cancer: updated clinical guidelines with an emphasis on germline CDH1 mutation carriers. J Med Genet 2015;52(6):361–74.
14. Wang K, Kan J, Yuen ST, et al. Exome sequencing identifies frequent mutation of ARID1A in molecular subtypes of gastric cancer. Nat Genet 2011;43(12): 1219–23.
15. Zang ZJ, Cutcutache I, Poon SL, et al. Exome sequencing of gastric adenocarcinoma identifies recurrent somatic mutations in cell adhesion and chromatin remodeling genes. Nat Genet 2012;44(5):570–4.
16. The Cancer Genome Atlas Research Network. Comprehensive molecular characterization of gastric adenocarcinoma. Nature 2014;513:202.
17. Cristescu R, Lee J, Nebozhyn M, et al. Molecular analysis of gastric cancer identifies subtypes associated with distinct clinical outcomes. Nat Med 2015;21(5): 449–56.
18. Wong SS, Kim KM, Ting JC, et al. Genomic landscape and genetic heterogeneity in gastric adenocarcinoma revealed by whole-genome sequencing. Nat Commun 2014;5:5477.
19. Ooi CH, Ivanova T, Wu J, et al. Oncogenic pathway combinations predict clinical prognosis in gastric cancer. PLoS Genet 2009;5(10):e1000676.
20. Lee J, Sohn I, Do IG, et al. Nanostring-based multigene assay to predict recurrence for gastric cancer patients after surgery. PLoS One 2014;9(3):e90133.

21. Lawrence MS, Stojanov P, Mermel CH, et al. Discovery and saturation analysis of cancer genes across 21 tumour types. Nature 2014;505(7484):495–501.
22. Wilson S, Fitzsimons M, Ferguson M, et al. Developing cancer informatics applications and tools using the NCI genomic data commons API. Cancer Res 2017; 77(21):e15–8.
23. Li X, Wu WK, Xing R, et al. Distinct subtypes of gastric cancer defined by molecular characterization include novel mutational signatures with prognostic capability. Cancer Res 2016;76(7):1724–32.
24. Chen K, Yang D, Li X, et al. Mutational landscape of gastric adenocarcinoma in Chinese: implications for prognosis and therapy. Proc Natl Acad Sci U S A 2015; 112(4):1107–12.
25. Kakiuchi M, Nishizawa T, Ueda H, et al. Recurrent gain-of-function mutations of RHOA in diffuse-type gastric carcinoma. Nat Genet 2014;46(6):583–7.
26. Siewert JR, Stein HJ, Feith M, et al. Histologic tumor type is an independent prognostic parameter in esophageal cancer: lessons from more than 1,000 consecutive resections at a single center in the Western world. Ann Surg 2001;234(3): 360–7 [discussion: 368–9].
27. Siewert JR, Ott K. Are squamous and adenocarcinomas of the esophagus the same disease? Semin Radiat Oncol 2007;17(1):38–44.
28. Kuwano H, Saeki H, Kawaguchi H, et al. Proliferative activity of cancer cells in front and center areas of carcinoma in situ and invasive sites of esophageal squamous-cell carcinoma. Int J Cancer 1998;78(2):149–52.
29. de Jonge PJ, van Blankenstein M, Grady WM, et al. Barrett's oesophagus: epidemiology, cancer risk and implications for management. Gut 2014;63(1):191–202.
30. Suh YS, Han DS, Kong SH, et al. Should adenocarcinoma of the esophagogastric junction be classified as esophageal cancer? A comparative analysis according to the seventh AJCC TNM classification. Ann Surg 2012;255(5):908–15.
31. Agrawal N, Jiao Y, Bettegowda C, et al. Comparative genomic analysis of esophageal adenocarcinoma and squamous cell carcinoma. Cancer Discov 2012; 2(10):899–905.
32. Shigaki H, Baba Y, Watanabe M, et al. PIK3CA mutation is associated with a favorable prognosis among patients with curatively resected esophageal squamous cell carcinoma. Clin Cancer Res 2013;19(9):2451–9.
33. Lin DC, Hao JJ, Nagata Y, et al. Genomic and molecular characterization of esophageal squamous cell carcinoma. Nat Genet 2014;46(5):467–73.
34. Katoh M. Function and cancer genomics of FAT family genes (review). Int J Oncol 2012;41(6):1913–8.
35. Rao RC, Dou Y. Hijacked in cancer: the KMT2 (MLL) family of methyltransferases. Nat Rev Cancer 2015;15(6):334–46.
36. Chung SM, Kao J, Hyjek E, et al. p53 in esophageal adenocarcinoma: a critical reassessment of mutation frequency and identification of 72Arg as the dominant allele. Int J Oncol 2007;31(6):1351–5.
37. Phillips WA, Russell SE, Ciavarella ML, et al. Mutation analysis of PIK3CA and PIK3CB in esophageal cancer and Barrett's esophagus. Int J Cancer 2006; 118(10):2644–6.
38. Dulak AM, Stojanov P, Peng S, et al. Exome and whole-genome sequencing of esophageal adenocarcinoma identifies recurrent driver events and mutational complexity. Nat Genet 2013;45(5):478–86.
39. Cancer Genome Atlas Research Network, Analysis Working Group: Asan University, BC Cancer Agency, et al. Integrated genomic characterization of oesophageal carcinoma. Nature 2017;541(7636):169–75.

40. Abrahao-Machado LF, Scapulatempo-Neto C. HER2 testing in gastric cancer: an update. World J Gastroenterol 2016;22(19):4619–25.
41. Bang YJ, Van Cutsem E, Feyereislova A, et al. Trastuzumab in combination with chemotherapy versus chemotherapy alone for treatment of HER2-positive advanced gastric or gastro-oesophageal junction cancer (ToGA): a phase 3, open-label, randomised controlled trial. Lancet 2010;376(9742):687–97.
42. Kankeu Fonkoua L, Yee NS. Molecular characterization of gastric carcinoma: therapeutic implications for biomarkers and targets. Biomedicines 2018;6(1) [pii:E32].
43. Young K, Chau I. Targeted therapies for advanced oesophagogastric cancer: recent progress and future directions. Drugs 2016;76(1):13–26.
44. Fuchs CS, Tomasek J, Yong CJ, et al. Ramucirumab monotherapy for previously treated advanced gastric or gastro-oesophageal junction adenocarcinoma (REGARD): an international, randomised, multicentre, placebo-controlled, phase 3 trial. Lancet 2014;383(9911):31–9.
45. Wilke H, Muro K, Van Cutsem E, et al. Ramucirumab plus paclitaxel versus placebo plus paclitaxel in patients with previously treated advanced gastric or gastro-oesophageal junction adenocarcinoma (RAINBOW): a double-blind, randomised phase 3 trial. Lancet Oncol 2014;15(11):1224–35.
46. Shah MA, Ramanathan RK, Ilson DH, et al. Multicenter phase II study of irinotecan, cisplatin, and bevacizumab in patients with metastatic gastric or gastroesophageal junction adenocarcinoma. J Clin Oncol 2006;24(33):5201–6.
47. Johnson DH, Fehrenbacher L, Novotny WF, et al. Randomized phase II trial comparing bevacizumab plus carboplatin and paclitaxel with carboplatin and paclitaxel alone in previously untreated locally advanced or metastatic non-small-cell lung cancer. J Clin Oncol 2004;22(11):2184–91.
48. Le DT, Durham JN, Smith KN, et al. Mismatch repair deficiency predicts response of solid tumors to PD-1 blockade. Science 2017;357(6349):409–13.
49. Muro K, Chung HC, Shankaran V, et al. Pembrolizumab for patients with PD-L1-positive advanced gastric cancer (KEYNOTE-012): a multicentre, open-label, phase 1b trial. Lancet Oncol 2016;17(6):717–26.
50. Ralph C, Elkord E, Burt DJ, et al. Modulation of lymphocyte regulation for cancer therapy: a phase II trial of tremelimumab in advanced gastric and esophageal adenocarcinoma. Clin Cancer Res 2010;16(5):1662–72.

Managing Squamous Cell Esophageal Cancer

Rishi Batra, MD, MBA[a], Gautam K. Malhotra, MS, MD, PhD[a], Shailender Singh, MD[b], Chandrakanth Are, MD, MBA[c],*

KEYWORDS

- Esophageal cancer • Squamous cell carcinoma • Foregut carcinoma

KEY POINTS

- Squamous cell carcinoma (SCC) accounts for about 90% of cases of esophageal cancer worldwide, with tobacco and alcohol use being significant risk factors, especially when used in combination.
- SCC arises from the stratified squamous epithelial lining of the esophagus because of repeated inflammation and mucosal damage of the esophagus, and is most commonly diagnosed with tissue biopsy during upper endoscopy (EGD).
- Treatment of lower-grade lesions (Tis and T1a) has moved to less invasive endoscopic procedures such as endoscopic mucosal resection or endoscopic submucosal dissection (ESD).
- NCCN guidelines recommend esophagectomy for locally advanced SCC (T1b-T4a or node-positive), but definitive chemoradiation remains an option for patients who decline surgery or are unfit for surgery.

INTRODUCTION

Each year, an estimated 455,800 new esophageal cancer cases occur worldwide, with 400,200 expected deaths. The global incidence burden and mortality is expected to continue to increase over time.[1] In the United States, the incidence of squamous cell carcinoma (SCC) has declined over the past 10 years, whereas the incidence of adenocarcinoma is on the increase. However, worldwide SCC still accounts for about 90% of esophageal cancer cases, with an estimated 398,000 worldwide.[2] Esophageal squamous dysplasia remains a major risk factor for developing SCC. Squamous cell carcinoma has a higher incidence in African Americans within North America and

Disclosure: The authors have nothing to disclose.
[a] Department of Surgery, University of Nebraska Medical Center, 983280 Nebraska Medical Center, Omaha, NE 68198, USA; [b] Internal Medicine, Division of Gastroenterology-Hepatology, 982000 Nebraska Medical Center, Omaha, NE 68198-2000, USA; [c] Department of Surgery, University of Nebraska Medical Center, 986880 Nebraska Medical Center, Omaha, NE 68198-6880, USA
* Corresponding author.
E-mail address: care@unmc.edu

remains a significant burden in East Asia, Africa, and South America.[1,3] The area extending from Northern Iran through the central Asia to North-Central China is often called the "esophageal cancer belt."[4,5] SCC has a male predominance with an average male-to-female ratio of 2.5. Studies have identified disparities in racial incidence, and the rate of SCC is 4.8-fold higher in African American men compared with white men.[1,2,6] As noted previously by Brown and colleagues,[6] tobacco use, alcohol use, low income status, and a diet lacking in raw fruits and vegetables are 4 risk factors that increase the risk of SCC in African Americans.

Given the current global burden of SCC and the expected growth in the future, a thorough understanding of the disease process is essential. This article will review the pathophysiology, risk factors, clinical presentation/diagnosis, and management of SCC. A systematic multi-disciplinary and methodical approach to patients with SCC is needed to provide high-quality care and to optimize outcomes.

RELEVANT ANATOMY/PATHOPHYSIOLOGY

The esophagus extends from the hypopharynx to the stomach and is approximately 25 cm in length. It is divided into 3 anatomic segments: cervical (lower end of pharynx to thoracic inlet), thoracic, and abdominal esophagus. A small percentage (5%) of SCC occurs in the cervical esophagus. Most SCC arise in the thoracic (middle) esophagus. In contrast, most adenocarcinomas of the esophagus develop in the distal esophagus. Squamous cell carcinoma arises from the stratified squamous epithelial lining of the esophagus because of repeated inflammation and mucosal damage of the esophagus. Early lesions presenting as "small polypoid excrescences, denuded epithelium, or plaques" are easily missed.[7] Many of these lesions begin with dysplastic changes with areas of "friability, a focal red area, erosion, plaque, or nodule" that can progress to more advanced lesions and invasive SCC.[8] The progression of SCC begins as esophageal squamous (epithelial) dysplasia, which transforms to carcinoma in situ, and subsequently develops into invasive carcinoma.[9] Tumor progression results in lesions that are ulcerated, friable, and necrotic. Lymphatic spread of disease occurs through the lamina propria, resulting in spread along the esophagus. Invasion into adjacent structures, including the trachea, results in fistula formation. Metastatic disease to the liver, bone, and lung occurs in approximately 30% of patients.[8]

Major risk factors for development of SCC include alcohol and tobacco use, and a synergistic effect has been reported with the combined use of both.[10] Alcohol and tobacco use accounts for 75% of cases in higher socioeconomic populations.[6,11] However, poor oral hygiene, deficient nutritional status, high levels of nitrosamines, and low intake of fruits and vegetables are thought to be dietary factors that may account for the increased incidence in Northern Iran and East Asia.[12-15] In addition, high-temperature beverages and foods have been associated with SCC secondary to thermal insult to the esophageal mucosa.[16,17] Injury to the esophageal mucosa, seen with caustic injury (such as Lye) and stricturing, increases the risk of SCC. Underlying esophageal dysmotility diseases, such as achalasia, can increase the risk of developing SCC by more than 16-fold.[18,19]

Multiple meta-analyses have been conducted, demonstrating an association between human papillomavirus (HPV) and esophageal SCC, with all studies noting HPV-16 to be the most prevalent strain present.[20,21] Li and colleagues[21] reported a significant association with a summarized odds ratio of 3.32 (95% CI, 2.26–4.87). However, a more recent analysis found an average prevalence of HPV in esophageal SCC was less than 40%.[22] Therefore, the exact role HPV in the pathogenesis of SCC is yet to be determined, as the evidence remains inconclusive.

CLINICAL PRESENTATION/EXAMINATION

Box 1 lists the signs and symptoms of SCC.

DIAGNOSTIC PROCEDURES

Routine screening for SCC is not currently recommended,[23] although it should be considered in those with known risk factors.[24] When clinical suspicion for SCC is present with any of the above signs or symptoms, upper gastrointestinal endoscopy (esophagogastroduodenoscopy [EGD]) is indicated for further work up and evaluation (**Fig. 1**). Given that many patients are asymptomatic on presentation, EGD may be indicated when significant risk factors alone exist and based on clinical suspicion. In the Linxian region of China, where SCC is prevalent, asymptomatic, high-risk SCC patients were screened with cytologic screening techniques using a deflated balloon and netting. This diagnostic method had a low sensitivity (14%–36%) for detection of SCC in patients with biopsy-confirmed diagnosis.[25,26]

As previously mentioned, early SCC may present as superficial plaques or ulcerations and a visible tumor may not be present. Traditional white light endoscopy remains the standard for upper endoscopy for identifying SCC lesions. However, newer endoscopic imaging techniques have been used to identify earlier lesions that may appear macroscopically normal.[26] Chromoendoscopy uses the application of Lugol's iodine to improve the visualization of SCC, and it has been shown that staining improves endoscopic detection and delineation of high-grade dysplasia and invasive squamous carcinoma.[27] Narrow-band imaging (NBI) is a novel imaging system that uses narrow-bandwidth filters in a red-green-blue sequential illumination system to identify early SCC (**Fig. 2**).[28,29] It is thought that NBI enhances chromoendoscopy without the use of dye agents.[30] Many of the other imaging modalities such as trimodal imaging, confocal fluorescence microscopy, elastic scattering spectroscopy, and optical coherence tomography have focused on the detection of adenocarcinoma of the esophagus given the increase in Western countries.[26] Unfortunately, limited data exist, demonstrating a significant benefit for detection over white light, and these methods have not been well studied in SCC. These new techniques are highly dependent on operator technique and interpretation and are therefore not currently universally recommended over white light endoscopy.

Box 1
Signs and symptoms of squamous cell carcinoma

Asymptomatic (early stages)

Dysphagia

Odynophagia

Unintentional weight loss

Retrosternal pressure, discomfort or a burning sensation

Epigastric pain

Persistent cough or hoarseness

Iron deficiency anemia from chronic gastrointestinal blood loss

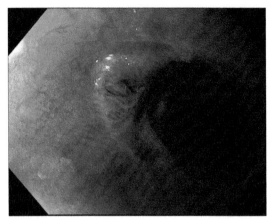

Fig. 1. Raised irregular lesion in the esophagus on esophagogastroduodenoscopy.

DIAGNOSIS

A histologic examination of tissue is needed for the diagnosis of SCC. Biopsies should be obtained of any suspicious areas or lesions. A diagnostic biopsy is obtained by upper endoscopy. Studies have shown that a single biopsy is confirmatory in over 90% of cases; obtaining up to 7 biopsies increases the accuracy to 98%.[31] If metastases are suspected, image-guided biopsy can also be obtained for tissue diagnosis. Following a tissue diagnosis, clinical staging can be conducted for assessment of locoregional disease as well as distant metastases. Staging includes the use of endoscopic ultrasound (EUS) for locoregional disease and the use of contrast-enhanced computed tomography of the neck, chest, and abdomen, and whole-body integrated fluorodeoxyglucose PET/computed tomography for distant metastases. The tumor, node, metastasis staging system of the combined American Joint Committee on Cancer/Union for International Cancer Control for esophageal cancer is the most commonly used worldwide (**Box 2**).

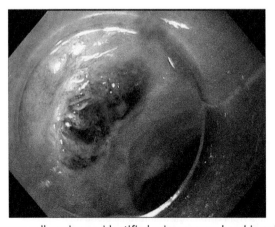

Fig. 2. Early squamous cell carcinoma identified using narrow-band imaging.

Box 2
Tumor, node, metastasis classification for esophageal squamous cell carcinoma

Primary tumor (T)

TX	Primary tumor cannot be assessed
T0	No evidence of primary tumor
Tis	High-grade dysplasia
T1	Tumor invades lamina propria, muscularis mucosae, or submucosa
T1a	Tumor invades lamina propria or muscularis mucosae
T1b	Tumor invades submucosa
T2	Tumor invades muscularis propria
T3	Tumor invades adventitia
T4	Tumor invades adjacent structures
T4a	Resectable tumor invading pleura, pericardium, or diaphragm
T4b	Unresectable tumor invading other adjacent structures, such as aorta, vertebral body, trachea, and so forth

Regional lymph nodes (N)

NX	Regional lymph node(s) cannot be assessed
N0	No regional lymph node metastasis
N1	Metastasis in 1–2 regional lymph nodes
N2	Metastasis in 3–6 regional lymph nodes
N3	Metastasis in 7 or more regional lymph nodes

Distant metastasis (M)

M0	No distant metastasis
M1	Distant metastasis

Histologic grade (G)

GX	Grade cannot be assessed: stage grouping as G1
G1	Well differentiated
G2	Moderately differentiated
G3	Poorly differentiated
G4	Undifferentiated: stage grouping as G3 squamous

Location (L)

X	Location unknown
Upper	Cervical esophagus to lower border of azygos vein
Middle	Lower border of azygos vein to lower border of inferior pulmonary vein
Lower	Lower border of inferior pulmonary vein to stomach, including gastroesophageal junction

Note: Location is defined by the position of the epicenter of the tumor in the esophagus.

MANAGEMENT OPTIONS AND OUTCOMES

As is true for most tumors, the treatment options for SCC vary by the disease stage at presentation. The American Joint Committee on Cancer staging system is widely accepted and used to stratify patients by the extent of disease progression and helps guide treatment decisions. Tumor staging for SCC is a complex matrix that takes into account the tumor size/depth of invasion, nodal status, presence of metastatic disease, tumor grade, and tumor location (see **Box 2**). Broadly speaking, tumors can be classified as superficial, localized, or unresectable/metastatic.

SUPERFICIAL SQUAMOUS CELL CARCINOMA

Superficial SCC is defined as cancer invading no deeper than the submucosal layer. Interestingly, the incidence of superficial esophageal cancer is increasing, which is thought to be because of increased surveillance.[32] As our understanding of superficial SCC has improved, and newer surgical/endoscopic techniques have emerged, we now have several treatment options available. Historically, even T1a mucosal lesions were treated with esophagectomy. The concern was inaccurate clinical staging and uncertainty of the nodal status. However, with advances in EUS, our ability to accurately stage patients has improved significantly. A large meta-analysis documented the sensitivity and specificity of EUS for detecting T1a lesions in the range of 85% and 87%, respectively. EUS was similarly effective for diagnosing T1b lesions with a sensitivity and specificity of 86% for both.[33] In addition endoscopic characteristics on imaging techniques such as NBI have been developed to accurately predict depth of invasion in SCC.[34] Several groups have also evaluated superficial SCC treated with esophagectomy to determine the incidence of nodal involvement. For Tis lesions, defined as high-grade dysplasia with malignant cells confined to the epithelium, several large studies have shown that there is minimal to no lymph node (LN) metastasis. Similarly, early T1a lesions have a low rate of LN metastasis, ranging from 0% to 9%.[35–38]

With our ability to accurately diagnose superficial SCC, and the low rate of LN involvement, there has been a shift in treatment preference from esophageal resection to less-invasive procedures such as endoscopic mucosal resection or endoscopic submucosal dissection (ESD) (**Fig. 3**). Endoscopic mucosal resection has now become the most common treatment used to treat T1a esophageal carcinoma in the United States.[39] In addition, there are several ablative techniques including photodynamic therapy, cryoablation, and radiofrequency ablation that can be used as definitive treatment of Tis lesions, or as adjuncts for T1a lesions. Esophagectomy, however, remains a viable treatment option for medically fit patients with early SCC.

Whereas endoscopic therapy has become more widely available and more commonly performed, it is important to note that these treatment options should only be offered to a very carefully selected patient population. As discussed above, Tis or T1a lesions have low rates of nodal involvement and are acceptable candidates. Furthermore, the lesion should ideally be solitary and small (ie, <2 cm) to facilitate complete R0 resection. Larger lesions often require piecemeal resection, which makes it difficult to assess the completeness of resection. Piecemeal resection is an established risk factor for recurrence.[40] One meta-analysis of ESD found a pooled R0 resection rate of 90% with smaller (<2.5 cm) lesions.[41] Finally, the lesion should have no evidence of lymphovascular invasion as these are associated with a high risk of nodal and distant metastasis, ranging from 41% to 47%, making them poor candidates for endoscopic resection (ER).[38,42] In contrast, T1a lesions without lymphovascular

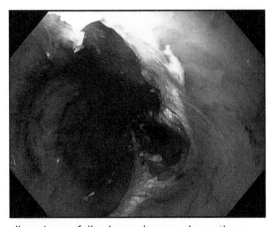

Fig. 3. Squamous cell carcinoma following endomucosal resection.

invasion have only a 0.7% 5-year rate of metastasis.[38] In addition, ulcerated or depressed lesions are often less amenable to ER because they have a tendency to invade deeper, and the inflammatory response can make it difficult to separate the mucosa from the submucosa.

In contrast to Tis and T1a lesions, all T1b tumors invading into the submucosa have high rates of LN involvement, ranging from 8% to 67% depending on the depth of sub-mucosal invasion.[35–38] Consequently, esophageal-preserving treatment options with endoscopic therapy exposes the patients to unacceptably high risk of local and distant recurrence and should be avoided.[43] These patients should undergo esopha-gectomy, preferably at a high-volume center.[44–46] The exception to this is for patients unfit for surgery, in whom ER with or without ablation can be considered. These pa-tients should also be considered for adjuvant chemoradiation if their lesions show ev-idence of poor prognostic features (lymphovascular invasion, poorly differentiated histology, positive margins, or size >2 cm).

LOCOREGIONAL SQUAMOUS CELL CARCINOMA

The management of locoregional esophageal cancer has evolved significantly over the last 20 years; this is especially true for esophageal SCC. Initially, localized disease was treated with surgery alone. However, the low cure rates and poor long-term survival prompted inclusion of systemic therapies and the multimodality treatment approaches that we currently use.[47–49] Today, upfront esophagectomy is reserved for T1 lesions (discussed above) and node-negative T2 lesions.

Early in the evolution of esophageal cancer treatment, it was recognized that esoph-agectomies were associated with significant morbidity and mortality[44–46] and 5-year survival rates ranging from 15% to 20%.[47–49] In this setting, radiation therapy (RT) was often used for local control. With modern radiation techniques including three-dimensional conformal radiation therapy and intensity-modulated radiation therapy, prospective randomized trials have shown similar 3- and 5-year overall survival rates for RT versus surgery alone.[50] However, surgery alone and RT alone offer only local control, and a significant percentage of treatment failure for locoregional disease is due to distant metastasis. This led to consideration of multimodal treatment strategies including systemic chemotherapy. Several trials have since been conducted to help determine the optimal treatment strategy (**Tables 1** and **2**). Two of the landmark trials are detailed below.

One of the early landmark trials, the RTOG 85-01 trial, compared RT alone (50 Gy) versus concurrent chemoradiotherapy (CRT) using infusional fluorouracil and cisplatin[51] (see **Table 2**). Surgery was not included in this study design. The trial was concluded prematurely when an interim analysis found a significant survival advantage for CRT. Five-year survival with CRT was found to be 27% compared with 0% for RT alone. Further analysis of the CRT arm revealed a significant reduction in both locoregional and distant failure rates. However, despite this, 46% of patients in the CRT arm still had local recurrence or persistent disease at 1 year, highlighting the need for surgery.

Following this, several trials began to compare neoadjuvant CRT with surgery alone. One of the largest was the Dutch CROSS trial, which was a prospective randomized trial of potentially resectable esophageal cancer comparing neoadjuvant CRT (with paclitaxel and carboplatin and concurrent 41.4 Gy RT) with surgery alone.[52] The study found statistically higher rates of R0 resection in the CRT group (92% versus 69%) and a 29% pathologic complete response rate. With a median follow-up of 32 months, the investigators found a significant improvement in the median overall survival for the

Table 1
Neoadjuvant chemoradiotherapy versus surgery alone

Trial, Year	N	SCC (%)	Treatment	Median Survival	3 y OS (%)	5 y OS (%)	pCR
Nygaard et al,[64] 1992	186	100	Surgery alone Neoadjuvant cisplatin and bleomycin Neoadjuvant RT Neoadjuvant CRT	Pooled survival			
Le Prise et al,[65] 1994	86	100	Neoadjuvant CRT (cisplatin, FU) Surgery alone		19.2 13.8		
Walsh et al,[59] 1996	113		Neoadjuvant CRT (cisplatin, FU) Surgery alone	16* 11*	32* 6*		25%
Bosset et al,[48] 1997	297	100	Neoadjuvant CRT (cisplatin) Surgery alone	18.6 18.6			
Burmeister et al,[66] 2005	256	37	Neoadjuvant CRT (cisplatin, FU) Surgery alone	22.2 19.3			9% adenoCA 27% SCC
Urba et al,[58] 2001	100	0	Neoadjuvant CRT (cisplatin, FU, vinblastine) Surgery alone	16.9 17.6	30 16		
Tepper et al,[67] 2008	56	23 27	Neoadjuvant CRT (cisplatin, FU) Surgery alone	53.8* 21.5*		39 16	40%
Van Hagen et al,[52] 2012	366	23	Neoadjuvant CRT (carboplatin, paclitaxel) Surgery alone	49* 24*	57* 44*	47* 34*	23% adenoCA 49% SCC

Abbreviations: CRT, chemoradiotherapy; FU, fluorouracil; N, nodal status; OS, overall survival; pCR, pathologic complete response; RT, radiation therapy; SCC, squamous cell carcinoma.
  * P<.05.

Table 2
Neoadjuvant chemoradiotherapy-based trials

Trial, Year	N	SCC (%)	Treatment	Median Survival	2 y OS (%)	3 y OS (%)	5 y OS (%)
Herskovic et al,[51] 1992	121	84 92	CRT (cisplatin + FU + 50 Gy) RT alone (64 Gy)	12.5* 8.9*	38* 10*		
Cooper et al,[68] 1999 (long-term data of above)	129	84 92	CRT (cisplatin + FU + 50 Gy) RT alone (64 Gy)				26* 0*
Minsky et al,[55] 2002	218		CRT (cisplatin + FU + 64.8 Gy) CRT (cisplatin + FU + 50 Gy)	13.0 18.1	31 40		
Conroy et al,[69] 2014	259		CRT (FOLFOX + 50 Gy) CRT (cisplatin + FU +50 Gy)	20.2 17.5		19.9 26.9	

* P<.05.

CRT arm (49.4 compared with 24 months in the surgery only group).[52] More recently published long-term follow-up data show a continued survival advantage in the preoperative CRT group, with a 5-year survival of 47% compared with 33% in the surgery only group.[53] These data support the use of a multimodal treatment paradigm using neoadjuvant chemotherapy with concurrent RT followed by surgical resection for suitable patients. However, a caveat of both the RTOG 85-01 and CROSS trials (and most esophageal cancer studies) is the inclusion of patients with both esophageal adenocarcinoma and SCC. Although initially treated as 2 diseases on the same spectrum, growing data suggest these are 2 very distinct disease processes with unique pathophysiology and treatment response.[54] This is demonstrated by the enhanced response to RT seen in SCC. Many studies have now looked into use of definitive CRT without surgery for SCC and found long-term survival in up to 27% of patients.[51,55–57] This is similar to long-term survival results seen in patients treated with neoadjuvant CRT followed by surgery,[58,59] neoadjuvant chemotherapy followed by surgery,[47,60] or surgery alone.[47,48]

With these data, several groups have investigated the use of definitive CRT compared with CRT + surgery in SCC.[61,62] Whereas both studies showed an improvement in locoregional control with the surgery group, neither was able to demonstrate improved survival. A Cochrane review of these 2 trials found that there was sufficient data and high-quality evidence that the addition of esophagectomy had no significant impact on survival.[63] Consequently, although the NCCN guidelines recommend esophagectomy for locally advanced SCC (T1b-T4a or node-positive), definitive chemoradiation remains an option for patients who decline surgery or are unfit for surgery.

UNRESECTABLE OR METASTATIC SQUAMOUS CELL CARCINOMA

Unfortunately, patients with locally advanced disease to the point of unresectability or for metastatic disease have limited treatment options. The goals of treatment in this patient population are often to palliate symptoms, improve quality of life, and prolong survival. Because of its efficacy for locoregional SCC, definitive CRT is the treatment choice for unresectable or metastatic disease. The hope for medically fit patients is for down-staging of their disease to transition them into a resectable candidate. There have been many randomized clinical trials evaluating various combinations of chemotherapy. Despite this, there is no globally accepted standard fist-line chemotherapy regimen. Currently in the United States, a platinum plus fluoropyrimidine doublet combination (eg, FOLFOX, CAPOX) is often used as first line treatment.

SUMMARY

Squamous cell carcinoma accounts for about 90% of cases of esophageal cancer worldwide, with significant burden in East Asia, Africa, and South America. Squamous cell carcinoma arises from the stratified squamous epithelial lining of the esophagus because of repeated inflammation and mucosal damage of the esophagus with most arising in the thoracic esophagus. Tobacco and alcohol are the significant risk factors for development of invasive disease. It is most commonly diagnosed with upper endoscopy (EGD). Treatment of lower-grade lesions (Tis and T1a) has moved to less invasive procedures such as ER via endomucosal resection or ESD. Several ablative techniques are now available such as photodynamic therapy, cryoablation, and radiofrequency ablation. Currently, NCCN guidelines recommend esophagectomy for locally advanced SCC (T1b-T4a or node-positive), whereas definitive chemoradiation remains an option for patients who decline surgery or are unfit for surgery.

REFERENCES

1. Malhotra GK, Yanala U, Ravipati A, et al. Global trends in esophageal cancer. J Surg Oncol 2017;115(5):564–79.
2. Arnold M, Soerjomataram I, Ferlay J, et al. Global incidence of oesophageal cancer by histological subtype in 2012. Gut 2015;64(3):381–7.
3. Rustgi AK, El-Serag HB. Esophageal carcinoma. N Engl J Med 2014;371(26): 2499–509.
4. Gholipour C, Shalchi RA, Abbasi M. A histopathological study of esophageal cancer on the western side of the caspian littoral from 1994 to 2003. Dis Esophagus 2008;21(4):322–7.
5. Tran GD, Sun X-, Abnet CC, et al. Prospective study of risk factors for esophageal and gastric cancers in the Linxian general population trial cohort in China. Int J Cancer 2005;113(3):456–63.
6. Brown LM, Hoover R, Silverman D, et al. Excess incidence of squamous cell esophageal cancer among US black men: role of social class and other risk factors. Am J Epidemiol 2001;153(2):114–22.
7. Hölscher A, Bollschweiler E, Schneider P, et al. Prognosis of early esophageal cancer. Comparison between adeno- and squamous cell carcinoma. Cancer 1995;76(2):178.
8. Dawsey SM, Wang GQ, Weinstein WM, et al. Squamous dysplasia and early esophageal cancer in the Linxian region of China: distinctive endoscopic lesions. Gastroenterology 1993;105(5):1333–40.
9. Kuwano H, Saeki H, Kawaguchi H, et al. Proliferative activity of cancer cells in front and center areas of carcinoma in situ and invasive sites of esophageal squamous-cell carcinoma. Int J Cancer 1998;78(2):149–52.
10. Prabhu A, Obi KO, Rubenstein JH. The synergistic effects of alcohol and tobacco consumption on the risk of esophageal squamous cell carcinoma: a meta-analysis. Am J Gastroenterol 2014;109(6):822–7.
11. Pandeya N, Olsen CM, Whiteman DC. Sex differences in the proportion of esophageal squamous cell carcinoma cases attributable to tobacco smoking and alcohol consumption. Cancer Epidemiol 2013;37(5):579–84.
12. Dar NA, Islami F, Bhat GA, et al. Poor oral hygiene and risk of esophageal squamous cell carcinoma in kashmir. Br J Cancer 2013;109(5):1367–72.
13. Van Rensburg SJ. Epidemiologic and dietary evidence for a specific nutritional predisposition to esophageal cancer. J Natl Cancer Inst 1981;67(2):243–51.
14. Schaafsma T, Wakefield J, Hanisch R, et al. Africa's oesophageal cancer corridor: geographic variations in incidence correlate with certain micronutrient deficiencies. PLoS One 2015;10(10):e0140107.
15. Pennathur A, Gibson MK, Jobe BA, et al. Oesophageal carcinoma. Lancet 2013; 381(9864):400–12.
16. Islami F, Boffetta P, Ren J-, et al. High-temperature beverages and foods and esophageal cancer risk - a systematic review. Int J Cancer 2009;125(3):491–524.
17. Wu M, Liu A-, Kampman E, et al. Green tea drinking, high tea temperature and esophageal cancer in high- and low-risk areas of Jiangsu province, China: a population-based case-control study. Int J Cancer 2009;124(8):1907–13.
18. Sandler RS, Nyrén O, Ekbom A, et al. The risk of esophageal cancer in patients with achalasia: a population-based study. J Am Med Assoc 1995;274(17): 1359–62.
19. Appelqvist P, Salmo M. Lye corrosion carcinoma of the esophagus. A review of 63 cases. Cancer 1980;45(10):2655–8.

20. Hardefeldt HA, Cox MR, Eslick GD. Association between human papillomavirus (HPV) and oesophageal squamous cell carcinoma: a meta-analysis. Epidemiol Infect 2014;142(6):1119–37.

21. Li X, Gao C, Yang Y, et al. Systematic review with meta-analysis: the association between human papillomavirus infection and oesophageal cancer. Aliment Pharmacol Ther 2014;39(3):270–81.

22. Petrick JL, Wyss AB, Butler AM, et al. Prevalence of human papillomavirus among oesophageal squamous cell carcinoma cases: systematic review and meta-analysis. Br J Cancer 2014;110(9):2369–77.

23. Wang KK, Wongkeesong M, Buttar NS. American gastroenterological association technical review on the role of the gastroenterologist in the management of esophageal carcinoma. Gastroenterology 2005;128(5):1471–505.

24. Tomizawa Y, Wang KK. Screening, surveillance, and prevention for esophageal cancer. Gastroenterol Clin North Am 2009;38(1):59–73.

25. Dawsey SM, Shen Q, Nieberg RK, et al. Studies of esophageal balloon cytology in Linxian, China. Cancer Epidemiol Biomarkers Prev 1997;6(2):121–30.

26. Bird-Lieberman EL, Fitzgerald RC. Early diagnosis of oesophageal cancer. Br J Cancer 2009;101(1):1–6.

27. Dawsey SM, Fleischer DE, Wang G-, et al. Mucosal iodine staining improves endoscopic visualization of squamous dysplasia and squamous cell carcinoma of the esophagus in Linxian, China. Cancer 1998;83(2):220–31.

28. Tajiri H, Matsuda K, Fujisaki J. What can we see with the endoscope? Present status and future perspectives. Dig Endosc 2002;14(4):131–7.

29. Gheorghe C. Narrow-band imaging endoscopy for diagnosis of malignant and premalignant gastrointestinal lesions. J Gastrointestin Liver Dis 2006;15(1): 77–82.

30. Kara MA, Peters FP, Rosmolen WD, et al. High-resolution endoscopy plus chromoendoscopy or narrow-band imaging in barrett's esophagus: a prospective randomized crossover study. Endoscopy 2005;37(10):929–36.

31. Graham DY, Schwartz JT, Cain GD, et al. Prospective evaluation of biopsy number in the diagnosis of esophageal and gastric carcinoma. Gastroenterology 1982;82(2):228–31.

32. Brown LM, Devesa SS. Epidemiologic trends in esophageal and gastric cancer in the United States. Surg Oncol Clin N Am 2002;11(2):235–56.

33. Thosani N, Singh H, Kapadia A, et al. Diagnostic accuracy of EUS in differentiating mucosal versus submucosal invasion of superficial esophageal cancers: a systematic review and meta-analysis. Gastrointest Endosc 2012;75(2):242–53.

34. Mizumoto T, Hiyama T, Oka S, et al. Diagnosis of superficial esophageal squamous cell carcinoma invasion depth before endoscopic submucosal dissection. Dis Esophagus 2018;31(7):1119–37.

35. Endo M, Yoshino K, Kawano T, et al. Clinicopathologic analysis of lymph node metastasis in surgically resected superficial cancer of the thoracic esophagus. Dis Esophagus 2000;13(2):125–9.

36. Fujita H, Sueyoshi S, Yamana H, et al. Optimum treatment strategy for superficial esophageal cancer: endoscopic mucosal resection versus radical esophagectomy. World J Surg 2001;25(4):424–31.

37. Shimada H, Nabeya Y, Matsubara H, et al. Prediction of lymph node status in patients with superficial esophageal carcinoma: analysis of 160 surgically resected cancers. Am J Surg 2006;191(2):250–4.

38. Yamashina T, Ishihara R, Nagai K, et al. Long-term outcome and metastatic risk after endoscopic resection of superficial esophageal squamous cell carcinoma. Am J Gastroenterol 2013;108(4):544–51.

39. Merkow RP, Bilimoria KY, Keswani RN, et al. Treatment trends, risk of lymph node metastasis, and outcomes for localized esophageal cancer. J Natl Cancer Inst 2014;106(7) [pii:dju133].

40. Ishihara R, Iishi H, Takeuchi Y, et al. Local recurrence of large squamous-cell carcinoma of the esophagus after endoscopic resection. Gastrointest Endosc 2008; 67(6):799–804.

41. Sun F, Yuan P, Chen T, et al. Efficacy and complication of endoscopic submucosal dissection for superficial esophageal carcinoma: a systematic review and meta-analysis. J Cardiothorac Surg 2014;9(1):78.

42. Eguchi T, Nakanishi Y, Shimoda T, et al. Histopathological criteria for additional treatment after endoscopic mucosal resection for esophageal cancer: analysis of 464 surgically resected cases. Mod Pathol 2006;19(3):475–80.

43. Akutsu Y, Uesato M, Shuto K, et al. The overall prevalence of metastasis in T1 esophageal squamous cell carcinoma: a retrospective analysis of 295 patients. Ann Surg 2013;257(6):1032–8.

44. Birkmeyer JD, Stukel TA, Siewers AE, et al. Surgeon volume and operative mortality in the United States. N Engl J Med 2003;349(22):2117–27.

45. Dimick JB, Wainess RM, Upchurch GR Jr, et al. National trends in outcomes for esophageal resection. Ann Thorac Surg 2005;79(1):212–6.

46. Begg CB, Cramer LD, Hoskins WJ, et al. Impact of hospital volume on operative mortality for major cancer surgery. J Am Med Assoc 1998;280(20):1747–51.

47. Kelsen DP, Ginsberg R, Pajak TF, et al. Chemotherapy followed by surgery compared with surgery alone for localized esophageal cancer. N Engl J Med 1998;339(27):1979–84.

48. Bosset J-, Gignoux M, Triboulet J-, et al. Chemoradiotherapy followed by surgery compared with surgery alone in squamous-cell cancer of the esophagus. N Engl J Med 1997;337(3):161–7.

49. Altorki N, Kent M, Ferrara C, et al. Three-field lymph node dissection for squamous cell and adenocarcinoma of the esophagus. Ann Surg 2002;236(2):177–83.

50. Sun XD, Yu JM, Fan XL, et al. Randomized clinical study of surgery versus radiotherapy alone in the treatment of resectable esophageal cancer in the chest. Zhonghua Zhong Liu Za Zhi 2006;28(10):784–7.

51. Herskovic A, Martz K, al-Sarraf M, et al. Combined chemotherapy and radiotherapy compared with radiotherapy alone in patients with cancer of the esophagus. N Engl J Med 1992;326(24):1593–8.

52. Van Hagen P, Hulshof MCCM, Van Lanschot JJB, et al. Preoperative chemoradiotherapy for esophageal or junctional cancer. N Engl J Med 2012;366(22): 2074–84.

53. Shapiro J, van Lanschot JJB, Hulshof MCCM, et al. Neoadjuvant chemoradiotherapy plus surgery versus surgery alone for oesophageal or junctional cancer (CROSS): long-term results of a randomised controlled trial. Lancet Oncol 2015;16(9):1090–8.

54. Wang K, Johnson A, Ali SM, et al. Comprehensive genomic profiling of advanced esophageal squamous cell carcinomas and esophageal adenocarcinomas reveals similarities and differences. Oncologist 2015;20(10):1132–9.

55. Minsky BD, Pajak TF, Ginsberg RJ, et al. INT 0123 (radiation therapy oncology group 94-05) phase III trial of combined-modality therapy for esophageal cancer:

high-dose versus standard-dose radiation therapy. J Clin Oncol 2002;20(5): 1167–74.

56. Crehange G, Maingon P, Peignaux K, et al. Phase III trial of protracted compared with split-course chemoradiation for esophageal carcinoma: Fédération Francophone de Cancérologie Digestive 9102. J Clin Oncol 2007;25(31):4895–901.

57. al-Sarraf M, Martz K, Herskovic A, et al. Progress report of combined chemoradiotherapy versus radiotherapy alone in patients with esophageal cancer: an intergroup study. J Clin Oncol 1997;15(1):277–84.

58. Urba SG, Orringer MB, Turrisi A, et al. Randomized trial of preoperative chemoradiation versus surgery alone in patients with locoregional esophageal carcinoma. J Clin Oncol 2001;19(2):305–13.

59. Walsh TN, Noonan N, Hollywood D, et al. A comparison of multimodal therapy and surgery for esophageal adenocarcinoma. N Engl J Med 1996;335(7):462–7.

60. Medical Research Council Oesophageal Cancer Working Group. Surgical resection with or without preoperative chemotherapy in oesophageal cancer: a randomised controlled trial. Lancet 2002;359(9319):1727–33.

61. Stahl M, Stuschke M, Lehmann N, et al. Chemoradiation with and without surgery in patients with locally advanced squamous cell carcinoma of the esophagus. J Clin Oncol 2005;23(10):2310–7.

62. Bedenne L, Michel P, Bouché O, et al. Chemoradiation followed by surgery compared with chemoradiation alone in squamous cancer of the esophagus: FFCD 9102. J Clin Oncol 2007;25(10):1160–8.

63. Vellayappan BA, Soon YY, Ku GY, et al. Chemoradiotherapy versus chemoradiotherapy plus surgery for esophageal cancer. Cochrane Database Syst Rev 2017;(8):CD010511.

64. Nygaard K, Hagen S, Hansen HS, et al. Pre-operative radiotherapy prolongs survival in operable esophageal carcinoma: a randomized, multicenter study of preoperative radiotherapy and chemotherapy. The second Scandinavian trial in esophageal cancer. World J Surg 1992;16:1104.

65. Le Prise E, Etienne PL, Meunier B, et al. A randomized study of chemotherapy, radiation therapy, and surgery versus surgery for localized squamous cell carcinoma of the esophagus. Cancer 1994;73:1779.

66. Burmeister BH, Smithers BM, Gebski V, et al. Surgery alone versus chemoradiotherapy followed by surgery for resectable cancer of the oesophagus: a randomised controlled phase III trial. Lancet Oncol 2005;6:659.

67. Tepper J, Krasna MJ, Niedzwiecki D, et al. Phase III trial of trimodality therapy with cisplatin, fluorouracil, radiotherapy, and surgery compared with surgery alone for esophageal cancer: CALGB 9781. J Clin Oncol 2008;26:1086.

68. Cooper JS, Guo MD, Herskovic A, et al. Chemoradiotherapy of locally advanced esophageal cancer: long-term follow-up of a prospective randomized trial (RTOG 85-01). Radiation Therapy Oncology Group. JAMA 1999;281:1623.

69. Conroy T, Galais MP, Raoul JL, et al. Definitive chemoradiotherapy with FOLFOX versus fluorouracil and cisplatin in patients with oesophageal cancer (PRODIGE5/ACCORD17): final results of a randomised, phase 2/3 trial. Lancet Oncol 2014;15:305.

Gastrointestinal Stromal Tumors of the Stomach and Esophagus

Lauren Theiss, MD, Carlo M. Contreras, MD*

KEYWORDS

• GIST • Stomach • Esophagus • Adjuvant • Neoadjuvant • Imatinib

KEY POINTS

• Molecular profiling is an important component of the work up and treatment of gastrointestinal stromal tumors (GISTs) and helps assess prognosis and select treatment options.

• Surgical resection is the mainstay of therapy for GISTs and can be done through open or minimally invasive approaches.

• Imatinib has been shown in many studies to benefit patients in the adjuvant setting.

• Patients with locally advanced and metastatic disease have also been shown to benefit from neoadjuvant or definitive imatinib therapy.

INTRODUCTION

Gastrointestinal stromal tumors (GISTs) overall represent a small percentage of gastrointestinal (GI) malignancies, but account for up to 80% of GI mesenchymal neoplasms.[1] These tumors can appear anywhere along the length of the GI tract including the stomach (60%), jejunum and ileum (30%), duodenum (4%–5%), rectum (4%), colon and appendix (1%–2%), and esophagus (<1%).[2] GISTs of the esophagus and esophagogastric junction have an incidence of 0.1 to 0.3 per million patients.[3] According to the SEER database, 6142 US patients were diagnosed with GISTs between 2001 and 2011.[4] However, the true incidence of GISTs is unknown owing to a historical lack of diagnostic criteria, and GISTs are likely much more common than data suggest. Recent studies have indicated that subclinical GISTs are likely more common in the general population than suspected, with 1 study identifying very small stromal tumors of the stomach in 22% of autopsies in adults greater than 50 years of age.[5] GISTs are more common in men than women and are also more common in older adults, with a mean age at diagnosis of 64 years.[4] The wide variety of anatomic

The authors have nothing to disclose.
Surgery, University of Alabama at Birmingham, Birmingham, AL, USA
* Corresponding author.
E-mail address: ccontreras@uabmc.edu

Surg Clin N Am 99 (2019) 543–553
https://doi.org/10.1016/j.suc.2019.02.012
0039-6109/19/© 2019 Elsevier Inc. All rights reserved.

locations and size of GISTs lead to a variety of clinical presentations, including but not limited to incidental detection, abdominal pain, GI blood loss, and intestinal obstruction. Although the complexities of GISTs lead to multiple clinical treatment scenarios, surgical resection remains the mainstay of therapy.

PATHOPHYSIOLOGY AND MOLECULAR PROFILING

GISTs originate from the interstitial cells of Cajal that reside in the myenteric plexus in the muscular layer of the GI tract. These cells regulate gut motility and serve as the pacemakers of the GI tract. Interstitial cells of Cajal are KIT, or CD117, positive, therefore staining for CD117 is diagnostic of GISTs in 75% to 80% of patients.[6] KIT is a gene that codes for a tyrosine kinase receptor named c-kit. C-kit is a proto-oncogene that, when activated, leads to unregulated proliferation of precursor cells. The platelet-derived growth factor receptor alpha is a proto-oncogene similar to c-kit, and mutations in this receptor similarly lead to formation of GISTs in 5% to 15% of cases. Both KIT and PDGFRA are found on chromosome 4. Mutations in each proto-oncogene cause constitutive phosphorylation of the receptor tyrosine kinase and lead to unregulated activation of downstream mediators. KIT mutations can be found on exons 9, 11, 13, or 17, while on the common PDGFRA gene mutations are found on exons 12, 14, or 18 (**Fig. 1**).[6] Thus, molecular profiling remains an important aspect of GIST identification and treatment.[7]

Approximately 10% of the GISTs that are not associated with KIT/PDGFRA mutations are termed wild-type GISTs (WT-GISTs) and are classified based on whether they are succinate dehydrogenase (SDH) deficient, or non-SDH deficient. SDH is an

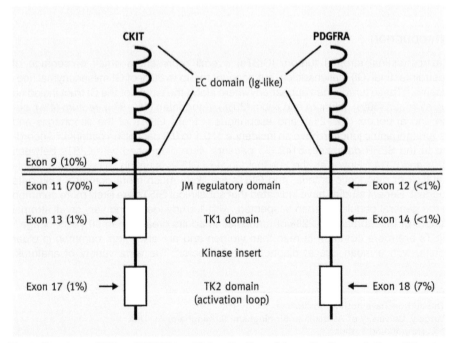

Fig. 1. Structure of KIT and PGDFRA, with localization of the activating mutations. EC, extracellular; JM, juxtamembrane; TK, tyrosine kinase. (*From* Tornillo, Luigi. Biology of gastrointestinal stromal tumour and mechanisms of imatinib resistance. Diagnostic Histopathology 2013;19(6): 203–10, with permission.)

important enzyme in the mitochondrial citric acid cycle as part of aerobic respiration. SDH loss leads to incomplete oxygen consumption and decreased energy production, leading the cell to develop a pseudohypoxic state as part of the Warburg effect. This results in cellular machinery driving neovascularization needed for tumor growth. The SDH-deficient tumors include patients with the Carney-Stratakis syndrome or the Carney triad. The Carney-Stratakis syndrome is characterized by GISTs and paraganglioma tumors due to germline mutations in the gene coding for the SDH enzyme.[8] This rare syndrome has an autosomal dominant mode of inheritance, with tumors arising in childhood and adolescence. Even more rare is the Carney triad, a nonhereditary disorder that commonly affects adolescent female patients. Hypermethylation of the SDH promoter causes downregulation of the enzyme, resulting in the development of GISTs, paraganglioma, and pulmonary chordomas. Neurofibromatosis type I is also an example of a non-SDH-deficient WT-GISTs.[9]

IMAGING, STAGING, AND PROGNOSIS

Imaging is essential in the diagnosis and staging of GISTs. Preoperative staging includes contrasted computed tomography (CT) evaluation of the chest, abdomen, and pelvis. Esophageal and esophagogastric junction GISTs are evident as solid masses on CT scan, often enhancing. Tumors are generally homogenous in character, with heterogeneity often indicating tumor necrosis or internal hemorrhage. The differential diagnosis for suspected GISTs on CT scan includes leiomyoma, leiomyosarcoma, congenital cyst, carcinoma, or neuroendocrine tumor.[10] The diagnosis of esophageal or gastric GISTs is often an incidental finding, but among symptomatic patients the most common findings are dysphagia, pain, reflux, and bleeding.[3] As GISTs arise as a submucosal tumor, the overlying mucosa on optical endoscopy will usually be normal. A standard endoscopic forceps mucosal biopsy will not adequately sample a GIST. Consequently, the preferred method for biopsy is an endoscopic ultrasound-guided needle biopsy, either a fine-needle aspirate or core. An enlarging submucosal GIST may grow either toward or away from the mucosal surface. Erosion through the mucosa is relatively common, which accounts for the capacity of these tumors to bleed. Erosion through the serosa is unusual, but secondary to trauma or intratumoral hemorrhage, esophageal and gastric GISTs can rupture into the peritoneal cavity resulting in hemoperitoneum and the acute onset of pain. Given the narrower viscus diameter, esophageal GISTs are typically not pedunculated as is common in the gastric location. Pedunculated GISTs can be either endophytic or exophytic. Thorough endoscopic and radiographic evaluation is essential as the surgical approach is shaped by these anatomic features.

Endoluminal biopsies are preferred over a percutaneous approach because of the small risk of tumor seeding along the tumor track. Spindle cells are the typical cytologic appearance of GISTs on fine-needle aspirate. At this point the differential diagnosis of spindle cells is quite broad, so the cellblock should be stained for CD117 and DOG-1 (discovered on GIST) to demonstrate a GIST.

The most common system used to stage GISTs is the American Joint Committee on Cancer (AJCC) 8th edition staging system released in January 2018. The AJCC establishes a difference in staging based on anatomic location (gastric vs nongastric GIST), and uses tumor size, lymph node involvement, distant metastases, and mitotic rate to stage sporadic GISTs in adult patients (see **Fig. 1**). The AJCC states that this staging system is not intended to be applied to pediatric or familial patients, or to syndromic patients with GISTs, because the tumor biology in these rare subsets is quite different than in sporadic cases.[11]

In addition to assigning stage, several scoring systems exist to assess the prognosis of GISTs after resection. Most include size of tumor, mitotic rate, and organ of origin. The Memorial Sloan-Kettering Cancer Center group created a nomogram using data from 127 patients that is used as a prognostic indicator for patients who underwent complete GIST resection without adjuvant therapy. This nomogram assigns points based on tumor size, mitotic index, and tumor site. It has been validated[12,13] to predict both 2- and 5-year recurrence survival. Other prognostic tools exist, such as the Armed Forces Institute of Pathology (AFIP) criteria, which have not been as extensively validated. The modified National Institutes of Health (NIH) criteria are commonly used by clinicians and use tumor site, size, mitotic rate, and intraoperative tumor rupture. The modified NIH criteria have also been validated and have been shown to be sensitive in predicting outcome in GISTs.[14–18]

In addition to tumor site, size, mitotic rate, and tumor rupture, complete surgical resection of disease is an important prognostic indicator for GISTs. R0 resection, or complete resection of all gross and microscopic disease as determined by pathologic review has been shown in numerous studies to be associated with improved local recurrence rate and overall survival.[19–21] Therefore, complete resection should be prioritized in the surgical approach to GISTs. GISTs with internal hemorrhage or necrosis can be quite friable and must be handled with care to prevent intraoperative rupture, which is essentially equivalent to a positive surgical margin.

OPEN VERSUS MINIMALLY INVASIVE RESECTION

Complete surgical resection is the gold standard treatment of GISTs. Tumors can be resected through open, thoracoscopic, laparoscopic, or robotic approaches. In 2015, Chen and colleagues[22] demonstrated no difference in long-term outcomes for patients who underwent laparoscopic versus open resection of gastric GISTs. However, the laparoscopic approach was associated with less blood loss, shorter postoperative length of stay, and a lower rate of perioperative complications. These findings indicate that a minimally invasive approach to resection of GISTs is both safe and appropriate.

The surgical approach to GIST resection should be determined by the surgeon, keeping in mind that key oncologic principles directly affect patient outcome and should be followed. Priority should be placed on a complete surgical resection of the tumor with negative margins. Care should be taken not to violate the tumor capsule and to remove the entire specimen without tumor spillage. If these principles can be safely followed, a laparoscopic approach is appropriate, especially for anatomically favorable areas such as the greater curve of stomach.

Surgical resection of esophageal GISTs poses a unique challenge due to the anatomic complexity of the esophagus and inability to perform simple wedge resection such as in the stomach. Tumors of the esophagus require complex surgical esophagectomy or tumor enucleation, and the preferred surgical approach is a topic still widely debated. Enucleation is generally considered acceptable for smaller tumors less than 5 cm however recent data suggest that enucleation is safe in tumors up to 6.5 cm.[23] Esophagectomy is usually reserved for larger tumors greater than 9 cm or tumors with high-risk features.[24,25] Regardless of tumor diameter, esophageal ulceration is generally considered an indication for esophagectomy, as enucleation is not technically feasible. Patient comorbidities and morbidity of the proposed operation should be considered in addition to tumor size and high-risk features when determining the appropriate approach to resection of esophageal GISTs.

Over the last 5 years, published reports of endoscopic resection of gastric GISTs have been increasing. These articles are generally small, retrospective, often include patients with GISTs as well as benign gastric lesions, and have limited data on long-term follow-up. One of the largest series included a total of 224 patients, 34% of whom had GISTs, and 54% of whom had a gastric tumor location.[26] Major complications including bleeding, perforation, or infection, occurring in nearly 10% of patients. Continued technologic advances in endoscopic luminal closure devices are likely to increase the application of this modality for esophageal and gastric GISTs. High quality studies are important in determining the patient and tumor characteristics that determine candidacy for an endoscopic resection approach.

ADJUVANT THERAPY

Some patients with GISTs require additional therapy beyond surgical resection. The molecular biology of GISTs is important in determining tumor response to adjuvant agents. Imatinib is a tyrosine kinase inhibitor (TKI) of c-kit that is the mainstay of medical therapy for GISTs with c-kit mutation. Generally, patients without c-kit or PDGFRA mutations are unlikely to respond well to imatinib therapy. However, some patients with WT-GISTs do indeed respond to therapy.

Imatinib is generally well tolerated by patients. The most common side effects are mild to moderate edema, nausea, diarrhea, myalgias, fatigue, and rash. Rarely, patients experience more serious side effects such as hepatotoxicity or myelosuppression, although myelosuppression is more common in patients undergoing imatinib therapy for chronic myeloid leukemia. Early concerns for cardiotoxicity have proven to be minimal, and most patients will tolerate imatinib therapy without significant side effects requiring cessation or pause in therapy.[27]

Adjuvant therapy for the treatment of GISTs has been well studied; however, the indications for imatinib and duration of treatment remain under debate. The ACOSOG Z9001 trial randomized patients with GIST greater than 3 cm in size to placebo or postoperative imatinib for 1 year after resection. Overall survival was unchanged however, recurrence-free survival was significantly higher in the imatinib arm, demonstrating a benefit to receiving adjuvant imatinib.[28] The SSG XVIII/AIO trial defined patients as high risk for GIST recurrence after resection based on modified NIH criteria (high mitotic index, size >5 cm, location outside of the stomach, and tumor rupture). Those patients defined as high risk for postoperative recurrence were randomized to 1 year or 3 years of adjuvant imatinib. Both recurrence-free survival and overall survival were higher in the group receiving 3 years of imatinib therapy. In 2012, Joensuu and colleagues[29,30] also reported that patients with GISTs categorized as high risk based on the NIH consensus criteria had improved recurrence-free survival and overall survival with 3 years of adjuvant imatinib, thus confirming a benefit in 3 years of adjuvant imatinib. Based on the above findings, as well as additional supporting data, the most recent National Comprehensive Cancer Network (NCCN) guidelines recommend adjuvant imatinib for at least 3 years in patients with high-risk GISTs based on tumor size, site, and location.[31] Two ongoing phase III trials are investigating longer courses of adjuvant imatinib therapy; the SSG XXII (NCT02413736) trial is evaluating 3 versus 5 years, and the ImadGist (NCT02260505) is evaluating 3 versus 6 years of therapy. The results of these trials are not expected for several years as both are currently accruing.

Adjuvant imatinib therapy has been shown to benefit patients in many clinical studies. Study populations frequently contain patients with gastric GISTs however, esophageal GISTs are less studied and often not included in study populations, indicating a need for further studies addressing the benefits of postoperative imatinib in these patients.[24] The increasing duration of adjuvant therapy is of interest from a health systems standpoint, as the annual cost of imatinib is approximately

$146,000.[32] At this cost, a Markov model was used to demonstrate that 3 years of adjuvant therapy falls within the commonly agreed upon threshold of $100,000 per quality-adjusted life-year threshold.[33]

Specific tumor mutations have been associated with information regarding sensitivity to specific TKI medication, the starting dose of that medication, and it may provide more individualized prognostic information. For this reason, request for mutation analysis should be considered for all patients with GISTs[31,34] (**Table 1**). In addition to the molecular subtypes shown in **Fig. 1**, tumors with the PDGRFA D842V mutation are unresponsive to imatinib and other standard TKIs, but may respond to dasatinib.[35]

LOCALLY ADVANCED AND METASTATIC DISEASE

The terms locally advanced and unresectable typically denote a tumor that cannot be removed without also resecting critical structures or organs that cannot otherwise be

Table 1
Molecular classification of GISTs

Genetic Type	Relative Frequency (%)	Anatomic Distribution	Notable Features
KIT mutation	77	–	–
Exon 8	Rare	Small bowel	
Exon 9	8	Small bowel, colon	Better responses higher-dose imatinib
Exon 11	67	All sites	Respond well to imatinib
Exon 13	1	All sites	Imatinib responsive
Exon 17	1	All sites	Many are imatinib sensitive
PDGFRA mutation	10	–	–
Exon 12	1	All sites	Sensitive to imatinib
Exon 14	<1	Stomach	Sensitive to imatinib
Exon 18 D842V	5	Stomach, mesentery, omentum	Imatinib resistant
Exon 18 other	1	All sites	Some but not all are imatinib sensitive
RTK-WT	13	All sites	–
RTK-WT/SDHB negative	–	–	–
SDH mutation (A/B/C/D)	~2	Stomach, small bowel	Carney-Stratakis syndrome
Carney triad	Rare	Stomach	Not heritable
Other (SDHA/B/C/D WT)	50–70 pediatric GIST but <2 GIST	Stomach only	Most pediatric and adults aged <30–40 y
RTK-WT/SDHB positive	–	–	–
BRAF V600E mutation	~2	All sites	–
RAS mutations	<1	Stomach	–
NF1-related	~1	Small bowel	Multiple lesions, rarely malignant
Other	5–10	All sites	Most RTK-WT GIST in adults >30 y

From Barnett CM, Corless CL, and Heinrich MC. Gastrointestinal stromal tumors: molecular markers and genetic subtypes. Hematology/Oncology Clinics 2013;27(5):871–88; with permission.

reconstructed. A patient might also be termed unresectable if they have a poor performance status and are not expected to survive the operation required to remove the tumor. In this sense, the definition of locally advanced or unresectable GIST is somewhat subjective, especially for patients with esophageal or gastric primary tumors. Considering the morbidity of esophagectomy, downstaging a tumor with the intent of being able to eventually perform a more limited or less morbid operation is a reasonable indication to discuss initiating neoadjuvant therapy. In contrast, an otherwise healthy patient with a small pedunculated gastric GIST and a single small liver metastasis should be considered for up-front surgical resection of both tumor sites followed by adjuvant therapy.

Three small prospective trials have evaluated outcomes for preoperative imatinib in patients with potentially resectable GISTs.[36–38] In aggregate they showed that a neoadjuvant approach was feasible in terms of drug toxicity, tumor shrinkage (median size reduction 34%), and morbidity of the combined treatment approach. In the Italian trial, neoadjuvant therapy downstaged all 15 of the study patients, resulting in a less morbid operation or complete surgical resection. In all 3 trials, neoadjuvant imatinib was continued for 2 years following surgical resection, which likely contributed to the favorable long-term survival reported in these studies. Although, among these 3 trials only 1 patient had a primary esophageal GIST, the results are generalizable.

Patients undergoing neoadjuvant therapy should continue until the optimal radiographic response has been achieved, with repeat CT scans every 8 to 12 weeks. The neoadjuvant approach should be terminated in patients who have evidence of progression, as the window of opportunity to perform a complete surgical resection can be slim. A potential drawback to a neoadjuvant approach is the theoretic risk of not being able to accurately assess the patient's need for adjuvant imatinib therapy. The preoperative biopsy, typically by endoscopic ultrasound, does not provide sufficient tumor volume to determine the mitotic index. The mitotic index observed in the surgical resection specimen may be confounded by the neoadjuvant imatinib. Because tumor size, anatomic location, and mitotic index affect the risk of postoperative recurrence, the decision to continue imatinib postoperatively may be clouded after neoadjuvant therapy.[31] At present, there are no nomograms or risk calculators that help assess the need for adjuvant therapy following the combination of neoadjuvant therapy and surgical resection.

The frequency of metastatic disease at presentation in patients with esophageal GISTs ranges from 17% to 48%.[3,39] Common sites for metastatic deposits include the peritoneal surface, liver, lungs, and bone. A thorough evaluation of the disease burden is essential to determine whether all tumor sites can be resected. Equally important is consideration of the perioperative risks and long-term consequences of complete resection. These elements should be discussed in a multidisciplinary forum to determine the optimal sequence of therapy.

Treatment recommendations for patients with locally advanced and metastatic GISTs should be based on tumor mutational analysis.[34,40] For susceptible patients, first-line therapy is imatinib. Patients with partial or high-grade esophageal or gastric obstruction because of tumor burden can still be considered for neoadjuvant imatinib therapy, as this medication can be dissolved in liquid for oral or enteral feeding tube administration.

The indications for pursuing second-line therapy include predicted tumor nonresponsiveness based on mutational analysis, toxicity to first-line therapy, or progression through first-line therapy. Second- and third-line agents are also orally administered TKIs, sunitinib and regorafenib, respectively. Dasatinib, another TKI was shown to have modest activity in patients with imatinib-resistant tumors, especially those patients with tumors expressing the proto-oncogene tyrosine-protein kinase Src.[41] Radiofrequency ablation or chemoembolization are options for patients with refractory liver metastasis. Palliative radiation therapy can be considered for the rare case of GIST metastasis to the bone.[31]

The surgical team should remain engaged with the patient undergoing systemic therapy for locally advanced or metastatic disease. Radiographic evidence of a favorable response should prompt reconsideration of surgical resection, either with curative or palliative intent. The typical interval for repeat cross-sectional imaging while receiving preoperative imatinib therapy is every 2 to 3 months, but an optimal response to imatinib therapy may take up to 6 months. Long-term therapy with any of the approved TKIs results in predictable drug resistance, so timely surgical intervention is crucial for achieving optimal long-term outcome. Imatinib is not associated with an increased risk of surgical complications, so preoperative therapy may be continued up to 24 hours before resection, and can be restarted in the adjuvant setting as soon as the patient has regained antegrade bowel function.

A retrospective review of 115 patients from a single institution in Oslo, Norway, indicated that oligometastatic disease, good performance status, and small tumor diameter were predictors of improved overall survival in comparison with patients with greater than 3 sites of metastatic GISTs.[42] Combined data from 2 American centers showed that patients who do not develop multifocal progressive disease while on TKIs for metastatic GISTs can be considered for cytoreductive surgery, although with significant morbidity.[43,44] Preclinical research suggests that immunotherapy may be appropriate for patients with GISTs.[45]

FOLLOW-UP AND SURVEILLANCE

Although limited data are available examining the optimal postoperative follow-up for GISTs, surveillance remains an important component of the management of resected, locally advanced, and metastatic GISTs. Patients should undergo routine history and physical every 3 to 6 months in addition to imaging for surveillance.[31] Contrasted CT scan of the abdomen/pelvis and MRI are both acceptable methods of imaging surveillance, as recurrence is rarely extra-abdominal. Joensuu and colleagues suggest that imaging frequency should be adjusted based on patient risk of recurrence as defined by prognostic indicators such as AFIP or the NIH consensus criteria. They recommend that patients with low-risk GISTs undergo abdominal CT scan annually for 5 years after resection. Patients with high-risk GISTs who have undergone adjuvant imatinib therapy should undergo surveillance more frequently once therapy is stopped, as risk of recurrence increases after therapy is discontinued. Joensuu and colleagues[46] recommend imaging every 6 months while receiving imatinib, every 3 to 4 months for the 2 years after therapy is stopped, and every 6 to 12 months for up to 10 years after resection. This surveillance schedule was not used in either of the major adjuvant randomized controlled trials, and is not currently included in NCCN guidelines. In summary, the surveillance schedule for a given patient should take into account the risk of recurrence, available treatments for recurrence, and risk of repeated radiation exposure on an individual basis.[31,47] Long-term surveillance for patients with GISTs is also important due to the observed risk of a second malignancy, observed in 19% of patients in a single-institution review. Incidental prostate and breast tumors were the most frequently observed events before GIST diagnosis, and renal and hematologic malignancies were the most frequently observed events after GIST diagnosis. GIST mitotic rate ≥ 5 per high power fields was identified as a risk factor for a second malignancy.[48]

SUMMARY

GISTs provide a unique challenge to the surgeon, because resection options vary greatly based on anatomic location. Beyond surgical treatment, neoadjuvant and adjuvant treatment of GISTs has been shaped by early molecular discoveries. However, treatment of GISTs remains a frequently studied topic with regard to duration of treatment, second-line therapies, and additional therapy options. GIST is a particularly fascinating malignancy that highlights the importance of a multidisciplinary treatment team.

REFERENCES

1. Miettinen M, Lasota J. Gastrointestinal stromal tumors – definition, clinical, histological, immunohistochemical, and molecular genetic features and differential diagnosis. Virchows Arch 2001;438(1):1–12.
2. Miettinen M, Lasota J. Gastrointestinal stromal tumors: pathology and prognosis at different sites. Semin Diagn Pathol 2006;23(2):70–83.
3. Briggler AM, Graham RP, Westin GF, et al. Clinicopathologic features and outcomes of gastrointestinal stromal tumors arising from the esophagus and gastroesophageal junction. J Gastrointest Oncol 2018;9(4):718–27.
4. Ma GL, Murphy JD, Martinez ME, et al. Epidemiology of gastrointestinal stromal tumors in the era of histology codes: results of a population-based study. Cancer Epidemiol Biomarkers Prev 2015;24(1):298–302.
5. Agaimy A, Wunsch PH, Hofstaedter F, et al. Minute gastric sclerosing stromal tumors (GIST tumorlets) are common in adults and frequently show c-KIT mutations. Am J Surg Pathol 2007;31(1):113–20.
6. Miettinen M, Lasota J. Gastrointestinal stromal tumors: review on morphology, molecular pathology, prognosis, and differential diagnosis. Arch Pathol Lab Med 2006;130(10):1466–78.
7. Lindsay T, Movva S. Role of molecular profiling in soft tissue sarcoma. J Natl Compr Canc Netw 2018;16(5):564–71.
8. Pasini B, McWhinney SR, Bei T, et al. Clinical and molecular genetics of patients with the Carney-Stratakis syndrome and germline mutations of the genes coding for the succinate dehydrogenase subunits SDHB, SDHC, and SDHD. Eur J Hum Genet 2008;16(1):79–88.
9. Andersson J, Sihto H, Meis-Kindblom JM, et al. NF1-associated gastrointestinal stromal tumors have unique clinical, phenotypic, and genotypic characteristics. Am J Surg Pathol 2005;29(9):1170–6.
10. Lewis RB, Mehrotra AK, Rodriguez P, et al. From the radiologic pathology archives: esophageal neoplasms: radiologic-pathologic correlation. Radiographics 2013;33(4):1083–108.
11. Jiao LR, Ayav A, Navarra G, et al. Laparoscopic liver resection assisted by the laparoscopic Habib Sealer. Surgery 2008;144(5):770–4.
12. Gold JS, Gonen M, Gutierrez A, et al. Development and validation of a prognostic nomogram for recurrence-free survival after complete surgical resection of localised primary gastrointestinal stromal tumour: a retrospective analysis. Lancet Oncol 2009;10(11):1045–52.
13. Chok AY, Goh BK, Koh YX, et al. Validation of the MSKCC gastrointestinal stromal tumor nomogram and comparison with other prognostication systems: single-institution experience with 289 patients. Ann Surg Oncol 2015;22(11):3597–605.
14. Agaimy A. Gastrointestinal stromal tumors (GIST) from risk stratification systems to the new TNM proposal: more questions than answers? A review emphasizing

the need for a standardized GIST reporting. Int J Clin Exp Pathol 2010;3(5): 461–71.

15. Sanchez Hidalgo JM, Rufian Pena S, Ciria Bru R, et al. Gastrointestinal stromal tumors (GIST): a prospective evaluation of risk factors and prognostic scores. J Gastrointest Cancer 2010;41(1):27–37.

16. Jang SH, Kwon JE, Kim JH, et al. Prediction of tumor recurrence in patients with non-gastric gastrointestinal stromal tumors following resection according to the modified National Institutes of Health criteria. Intest Res 2014;12(3):229–35.

17. Joensuu H, Vehtari A, Riihimaki J, et al. Risk of recurrence of gastrointestinal stromal tumour after surgery: an analysis of pooled population-based cohorts. Lancet Oncol 2012;13(3):265–74.

18. Rutkowski P, Bylina E, Wozniak A, et al. Validation of the Joensuu risk criteria for primary resectable gastrointestinal stromal tumour - the impact of tumour rupture on patient outcomes. Eur J Surg Oncol 2011;37(10):890–6.

19. Ng EH, Pollock RE, Munsell MF, et al. Prognostic factors influencing survival in gastrointestinal leiomyosarcomas. Implications for surgical management and staging. Ann Surg 1992;215(1):68–77.

20. DeMatteo RP, Lewis JJ, Leung D, et al. Two hundred gastrointestinal stromal tumors: recurrence patterns and prognostic factors for survival. Ann Surg 2000; 231(1):51.

21. Aparicio T, Boige V, Sabourin JC, et al. Prognostic factors after surgery of primary resectable gastrointestinal stromal tumours. Eur J Surg Oncol 2004;30(10): 1098–103.

22. Chen K, Zhou YC, Mou YP, et al. Systematic review and meta-analysis of safety and efficacy of laparoscopic resection for gastrointestinal stromal tumors of the stomach. Surg Endosc 2015;29(2):355–67.

23. Robb WB, Bruyere E, Amielh D, et al. Esophageal gastrointestinal stromal tumor: is tumoral enucleation a viable therapeutic option? Ann Surg 2015;261(1):117–24.

24. Hihara J, Mukaida H, Hirabayashi N. Gastrointestinal stromal tumor of the esophagus: current issues of diagnosis, surgery and drug therapy. Transl Gastroenterol Hepatol 2018;3:6.

25. Duffaud F, Meeus P, Bertucci F, et al. Patterns of care and clinical outcomes in primary oesophageal gastrointestinal stromal tumours (GIST): a retrospective study of the French Sarcoma Group (FSG). Eur J Surg Oncol 2017;43(6):1110–6.

26. He G, Wang J, Chen B, et al. Feasibility of endoscopic submucosal dissection for upper gastrointestinal submucosal tumors treatment and value of endoscopic ultrasonography in pre-operation assess and post-operation follow-up: a prospective study of 224 cases in a single medical center. Surg Endosc 2016;30(10):4206–13.

27. Ben Ami E, Demetri GD. A safety evaluation of imatinib mesylate in the treatment of gastrointestinal stromal tumor. Expert Opin Drug Saf 2016;15(4):571–8.

28. Corless CL, Ballman KV, Antonescu CR, et al. Pathologic and molecular features correlate with long-term outcome after adjuvant therapy of resected primary GI stromal tumor: the ACOSOG Z9001 trial. J Clin Oncol 2014;32(15):1563–70.

29. Joensuu H, Eriksson M, Sundby Hall K, et al. Adjuvant imatinib for high-risk GI stromal tumor: analysis of a randomized trial. J Clin Oncol 2016;34(3):244–50.

30. Joensuu H, Eriksson M, Sundby Hall K, et al. One vs three years of adjuvant imatinib for operable gastrointestinal stromal tumor: a randomized trial. JAMA 2012; 307(12):1265–72.

31. Network NCC. Soft tissue sarcoma, vol. 2, 2018. Available at: https://www.nccn. org/professionals/physician_gls/pdf/sarcoma.pdf. Accessed November 21, 2018.

32. Kantarjian H. The arrival of generic imatinib into the U.S. market: an educational event. The ASCO Post 2016;(7):110–1.
33. Sanon M, Taylor DC, Parthan A, et al. Cost-effectiveness of 3-years of adjuvant imatinib in gastrointestinal stromal tumors (GIST) in the United States. J Med Econ 2013;16(1):150–9.
34. von Mehren M, Joensuu H. Gastrointestinal stromal tumors. J Clin Oncol 2018; 36(2):136–43.
35. Dewaele B, Wasag B, Cools J, et al. Activity of dasatinib, a dual SRC/ABL kinase inhibitor, and IPI-504, a heat shock protein 90 inhibitor, against gastrointestinal stromal tumor-associated PDGFRAD842V mutation. Clin Cancer Res 2008; 14(18):5749–58.
36. McAuliffe JC, Hunt KK, Lazar AJ, et al. A randomized, phase II study of preoperative plus postoperative imatinib in GIST: evidence of rapid radiographic response and temporal induction of tumor cell apoptosis. Ann Surg Oncol 2009;16(4):910–9.
37. Fiore M, Palassini E, Fumagalli E, et al. Preoperative imatinib mesylate for unresectable or locally advanced primary gastrointestinal stromal tumors (GIST). Eur J Surg Oncol 2009;35(7):739–45.
38. Eisenberg BL, Harris J, Blanke CD, et al. Phase II trial of neoadjuvant/adjuvant imatinib mesylate (IM) for advanced primary and metastatic/recurrent operable gastrointestinal stromal tumor (GIST): early results of RTOG 0132/ACRIN 6665. J Surg Oncol 2009;99(1):42–7.
39. Kukar M, Kapil A, Papenfuss W, et al. Gastrointestinal stromal tumors (GISTs) at uncommon locations: a large population based analysis. J Surg Oncol 2015; 111(6):696–701.
40. Zeichner SB, Goldstein DA, Kohn C, et al. Cost-effectiveness of precision medicine in gastrointestinal stromal tumor and gastric adenocarcinoma. J Gastrointest Oncol 2017;8(3):513–23.
41. Schuetze SM, Bolejack V, Thomas DG, et al. Association of dasatinib with progression-free survival among patients with advanced gastrointestinal stromal tumors resistant to imatinib. JAMA Oncol 2018;4(6):814–20.
42. Hompland I, Bruland OS, Holmebakk T, et al. Prediction of long-term survival in patients with metastatic gastrointestinal stromal tumor: analysis of a large, single-institution cohort. Acta Oncol 2017;56(10):1317–23.
43. Fairweather M, Cavnar MJ, Li GZ, et al. Prediction of morbidity following cytoreductive surgery for metastatic gastrointestinal stromal tumour in patients on tyrosine kinase inhibitor therapy. Br J Surg 2018;105(6):743–50.
44. Fairweather M, Balachandran VP, Li GZ, et al. Cytoreductive surgery for metastatic gastrointestinal stromal tumors treated with tyrosine kinase inhibitors: a 2-institutional analysis. Ann Surg 2018;268(2):296–302.
45. Pantaleo MA, Indio V, Tarantino G, et al. Immune microenvironment profiling of gastrointestinal stromal tumors (GIST). J Clin Oncol 2018;36(15_suppl):11534.
46. Joensuu H, Martin-Broto J, Nishida T, et al. Follow-up strategies for patients with gastrointestinal stromal tumour treated with or without adjuvant imatinib after surgery. Eur J Cancer 2015;51(12):1611–7.
47. Nishida T, Blay JY, Hirota S, et al. The standard diagnosis, treatment, and follow-up of gastrointestinal stromal tumors based on guidelines. Gastric Cancer 2016; 19(1):3–14.
48. Hechtman JF, DeMatteo R, Nafa K, et al. Additional primary malignancies in patients with gastrointestinal stromal tumor (GIST): a clinicopathologic study of 260 patients with molecular analysis and review of the literature. Ann Surg Oncol 2015;22(8):2633–9.

Palliative Management of Gastric and Esophageal Cancer

Alison L. Halpern, MD, Martin D. McCarter, MD*

KEYWORDS

- Palliative care • Gastric cancer • Esophageal cancer • Endoscopic therapy
- Dysphagia • Malignant obstruction

KEY POINTS

- Patients with esophageal or gastric cancer presenting with metastatic disease are not candidates for curative surgical therapy and treatment options often focus on palliation.
- Many endoscopic techniques are effective in treating dysphagia or obstruction.
- Nutritional access is a common need in patients with advanced esophageal and gastric cancer and may be obtained via endoscopic or percutaneous procedures.
- Owing to the mortality and morbidity associated with surgery in patients with a short life expectancy, surgical palliation has fallen out of favor when compared with local endoscopic therapies.
- Surgery may be necessary in patients presenting with perforation secondary to their disease or other symptomatology that cannot be controlled by less invasive interventions alone.

INTRODUCTION

In the United States, there are more than 17,000 patients diagnosed with esophageal cancer annually and more than 26,000 new diagnoses of gastric cancer annually. Overall, patients presenting with esophageal cancer have an estimated 5-year survival of 18.8% and patients presenting with gastric cancer have an estimated 5-year survival of 30.6%. For patients presenting with distant disease there is an approximate 5-year survival of 5% for both diseases.[1,2] Surgical resection in combination with chemotherapy or chemoradiotherapy is the mainstay of curative therapy in both diseases. However, many patients present with unresectable disease at diagnosis or may progress to unresectable disease throughout their clinical course. For these

The authors have nothing to disclose.
Department of Surgery, Division of Surgical Oncology, University of Colorado School of Medicine, 12631 East 17th Avenue, C302, Aurora, CO 80045, USA
* Corresponding author.
E-mail address: martin.mccarter@ucdenver.edu

patients, palliative chemoradiotherapy is the standard of care if patients have an appropriate performance status. Palliative chemoradiotherapy is recommended to extend progression-free survival, but in this cohort of patients with advanced disease, it is highly likely that palliation of symptoms rather than cure will become a focus of treatment.

Given the similar anatomic location of both diseases, there are common symptoms or complications in patients presenting with advanced gastric and esophageal cancer. These complications include dysphagia, obstruction, bleeding, nutritional issues, and pain, among others. The treatment of these issues in the patient receiving palliative care with gastric or esophageal cancer requires a multidisciplinary team to include endoluminal therapy, chemotherapy, radiotherapy, pain management, and surgery. The interventions provided should always reflect the patient's goals of care.

Unknown to many, the phrase palliative care was actually first termed by a surgeon, Balfour Mount, MD, to describe a multidisciplinary, comprehensive care team focused on patient-centered goals and symptom relief in the dying patient.[3] One of the key tenets of palliative care includes a patient-centered approach, where treatments are focused on the patient's specific goals of care, including the relief of symptoms, even if the interventions are not life prolonging.

STAGING DETERMINES RESECTABILITY IN ESOPHAGEAL AND GASTRIC CANCER

Patients presenting with gastric or esophageal cancer should receive a multidisciplinary evaluation of their disease. Patients should undergo thorough clinical staging related to their specific disease. According to the National Comprehensive Cancer Network guidelines, patients with esophageal or gastric cancer presenting with M1 disease according to the Tumor Node Metastasis (TNM) Classification of Malignant Tumors are generally considered unresectable.[4,5] Attempts at curative surgery are not recommended for these patients and, thus, they are generally advised to undergo palliative chemoradiotherapy or systemic therapy if they have an appropriate performance score (**Table 1**).

Palliation of Symptoms in Advanced Gastric and Esophageal Cancer

If a patient with esophageal or gastric cancer has been confirmed as not a candidate for surgery or has progressed to failure through traditional therapy, it is appropriate to focus on symptom control.[6] Similar to the multidisciplinary nature of curative cancer therapy, a palliative symptom-based approach to therapy should also include a multidisciplinary team.[7]

Dysphagia and Obstruction

It is exceptionally common for patients with advanced gastric and esophageal cancer to present with obstructive symptoms from gastric and esophageal cancers that occlude the lumen of the affected organ. Patients may present with varying degrees of dysphagia or obstruction and quantifying their symptoms with either the Dysphagia Grading Score or the Gastric Outlet Obstruction Score can be useful to determine the efficacy of intervention.[8,9] Herein we discuss treatment options to palliate dysphagia and obstruction (**Boxes 1 and 2; Fig. 1**).

Palliation of Dysphagia and Obstruction: Endoscopic Dilation

Esophageal or gastric dilation at the site of an obstruction caused by a tumor is performed via upper endoscopy, using a pneumatic balloon or wire-covered bougie.[10] Dilation can provide near immediate relief of dysphagia and obstructive symptoms,

Table 1
The Karnofsky and ECOG performance scores

Karnofsky Status	Karnofsky Grade	ECOG Grade	ECOG Status
Normal, no complaints	100	0	Fully active, able to carry on all predisease activities without restriction
Able to carry on normal activities; minor signs or symptoms of disease	90	1	Restricted in physically strenuous activity but ambulatory and able to carry out work of a light or sedentary nature, for example, light house work, office work
Normal activity with effort	80	1	Restricted in physically strenuous activity but ambulatory and able to carry out work of a light or sedentary nature, for example, light house work, office work
Care for self; unable to carry on normal activity or to do active work	70	2	Ambulatory and capable of all self-care, but unable to carry out any work activities; up and about more than 50% of waking hours
Requires occasional assistance, but able to care for most of her or his needs	60	2	Ambulatory and capable of all self-care, but unable to carry out any work activities; up and about more than 50% of waking hours
Requires considerable assistance and frequent medical care	50	3	Capable of only limited self-care, confined to bed or chair more than 50% of waking hours
Disabled; requires special care and assistance	40	3	Capable of only limited self-care, confined to bed or chair more than 50% of waking hours
Severely disabled; hospitalization indicated although death is not imminent	30	4	Completely disabled; cannot carry on any self-care; totally confined to bed or chair
Very sick; hospitalization necessary; active supportive treatment necessary	20	4	Completely disabled; cannot carry on any self-care; totally confined to bed or chair
Moribund	10	4	Completely disabled; cannot carry on any self-care; totally confined to bed or chair
Dead	0	5	Dead

Abbreviation: ECOG, Eastern Cooperative Oncology Group.
Performance scores are used when determining if a patient is an appropriate candidate for therapy.
From Oken MM, Creech RH, Tormey DC, et al. Toxicity and response criteria of the Eastern Cooperative Oncology Group. Am J Clin Oncol 1982;5: 651, with permission.

although the relief is not often durable in the setting of malignant obstruction **(Fig. 2)**.[8,10,11]

Palliation of Dysphagia and Obstruction: Endoscopic Stenting

Esophageal or gastric stenting at the site of an obstruction caused by a tumor is also performed via upper endoscopy, often after dilation to an esophageal diameter of

---

Box 1
The Dysphagia Grading System, used to assess patient's degree of dysphagia symptoms

Grade 0 = Able to eat normal diet. No dysphagia reported.

Grade 1 = Able to swallow some solid foods.

Grade 2 = Able to swallow only semisolid or soft foods.

Grade 3 = Able to swallow liquids only.

Grade 4 = Unable to swallow anything.

Data from Knyrim K, Wagner HJ, Bethge N, et al. A controlled trial of an expansile metal stent for palliation of esophageal obstruction due to inoperable cancer. N Engl J Med 1993;329:1302–7.

---

approximately 1 cm. Endoscopic stenting often provides durable relief of obstructive symptoms secondary to tumor. Self-expanding metal stents came into existence in the 1990s with the growing capabilities of endoluminal therapy. In addition to self-expanding metal stents, there are also commercially available plastic stents as well as covered versions of both plastic and metal stents. The advantage of a covered stent is that it resists tumor ingrowth, and the disadvantage of a covered stent is that it has a higher likelihood of migration.[10,12,13]

Patients who undergo esophageal stenting for malignant esophageal cancer generally experience a significant improvement in their dysphagia symptoms, with more than 95% of patients able to tolerate liquids (dysphagia grade $\geq$3) after stent placement (**Figs. 3** and **4**).[11,14–19] Although stenting is more common in the setting of malignant esophageal obstruction, it also has been used to treat gastric outlet obstruction as a result of gastric cancer. A recent analysis concluded that gastroduodenal stent placement was feasible, effective, and safe in the treatment of malignant gastric outlet obstruction.[20] Gastric outlet obstruction stenting shares the same benefits and risks as esophageal stenting; it provides near immediate relief of symptoms, but may be complicated rarely by perforation, a persistent pressure sensation for patients, and stents may migrate or be reobstructed by tumor progression. When compared with other palliative measures for gastric outlet obstruction, patients who received stents had faster relief of symptoms and shorter hospital stays than patients who underwent surgical palliation of obstruction.[13,21–24]

Palliation of Dysphagia: Alternate Modalities

Although endoscopic dilation and stenting of gastric and esophageal malignancies is fairly common, other modalities of local therapy may work independently or, more

---

Box 2
The Gastric Outlet Obstruction Scoring System, used to assess patient's degree of obstructive symptoms

Grade 0 = No oral intake.

Grade 1 = Liquids only.

Grade 2 = Soft solids.

Grade 3 = Low residue or full diet.

Data from Adler DG, Baron TH. Endoscopic palliation of malignant gastric outlet obstruction using self-expanding metal stents: experience in 36 patients. Am J Gastroenterol 2002;97:72–8.

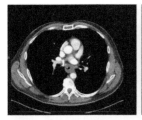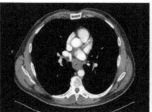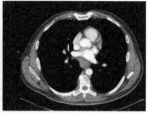

Fig. 1. Computed tomography imaging showing serial images of a middle third esophageal mass that completely obstructs the lumen in a patient presenting with progressive dysphagia and obstruction.

often, in conjunction with dilation and stenting. It should be noted that all endoluminal ablative therapies as well as stents carry the risk of perforation, formation of esophageal fistulas, recurrence of symptoms, and other therapy-specific complications.

Endoluminal Brachytherapy

This technique involves the endoscopic introduction of a radioactive source into the tumor. By specifically targeting the tumor itself from an endoscopic approach, the tumor itself receives a high dose of radiotherapy with a relatively small involvement of the surrounding healthy tissues.[25] Brachytherapy is delivered weekly via endoscopy during a 3- to 8-week treatment course.[26,27] This therapy confers a robust response rate of up to 70% for dysphagia symptoms, but the symptom relief has been reported as brief, lasting an average of 2.5 months. In brachytherapy, the pitfalls include the need for multiple treatments as well as the risk of esophagitis, stricture, and fistula. However, a recent study of patients with primary, posttreatment persistent or recurrent esophageal cancer demonstrated a more than 50% pathologic complete response in patients who received endoluminal high-dose rate brachytherapy and this therapy notably can still be used after tumor progression for patients who have already received external beam radiotherapy, so it remains a useful tool in the palliation of advanced disease.[25–27]

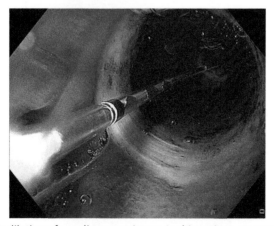

Fig. 2. Endoscopic dilation of a malignant stricture. In this patient, an upper endoscopy was performed, and a malignant stricture was apparent. A dilator was passed through the endoscope and the malignant stricture and serial balloon dilations were performed until the stricture was improved.

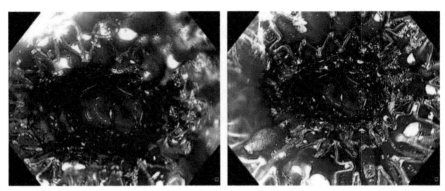

Fig. 3. A self-expanding metal stent is seen in the esophagus of a patient with esophageal cancer who presented with grade 4 dysphagia symptoms before dilation and stenting. After the procedure, he was able to easily tolerate liquids (grade 3 dysphagia).

Photodynamic Therapy

Photodynamic therapy involves the parenteral administration of a systemic photosensitizer followed by the administration of locally directed light. The photosensitizer is preferentially taken up by tumor cells and, when the specific wavelength of light required by the specific photosensitizer is applied to the tumor via an endoscope, a

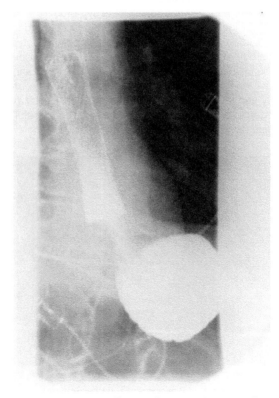

Fig. 4. Esophagram demonstrating a self-expanding metal stent in the middle third of the esophagus with successful passage of contrast through the stent and into the stomach.

photooxidative reaction occurs and cell death follows. The phototherapy is typically applied 48 to 72 hours after the administration of the photosensitizing agent. Repeat endoscopy is performed 48 to 72 hours after the initial phototherapy to assess tumor response, debride tissue, and potentially apply repeat phototherapy. Phototherapy remains one of the less popular endoscopic ablative therapies owing to its limited efficacy data and the fact that patients receiving photodynamic therapy must avoid sunlight after receiving the systemic photosensitizer.[10,28,29]

Laser Therapy

Local laser therapy to address obstruction includes treatment with high-energy lasers, such as the Nd:YAG laser. This therapy works by vaporizing tumor tissue through a high-intensity laser light beam. Through an endoscope, a laser beam is directed at the obstructing esophageal or gastric tumor, approximately 1 cm away from the tumor. The laser then delivers energy to the tumor, which in turn creates coagulation and vaporization of the tumor tissue. Early studies of the Nd:YAG laser demonstrated a rapid improvement in dysphagia scores in patients undergoing laser therapy.[30–32] It has been shown that patients with short segment bulky tumors benefit more so from this therapy than those with longer segments of obstructing tumor.[30,33,34] The average duration of symptom improvement after laser ablative therapy has been reported to be 4 weeks and can be a useful component of local therapy.[35]

Endoscopic Alcohol Injection

Endoscopic alcohol injection, otherwise known as ethanol-induced tumor necrosis, is a simple endoscopic procedure that involves the local injection of pure ethanol via sclerosing needles into the obstructing tumor. Regarding the procedure, up to 10 mL of pure ethanol is injected in 1-mL aliquots circumferentially into the tumor at the level of the obstruction.[36,37] This procedure requires less technology than laser ablating techniques or endoscopic stenting. The average duration of symptom improvement after endoscopic alcohol injection is similar to laser ablative therapy at approximately 4 weeks to recurrence of symptoms.[38]

Endoscopic Injection of Chemotherapy

In addition to the endoscopic injection of alcohol as an ablative agent, another modality of local therapy for esophageal or gastric cancer is the endoscopic injection of chemotherapy for esophageal and gastric tumors. In this procedure, a chemotherapy (most commonly 5-fluorouracil, but occasionally mitomycin C) is injected into the tumor.[39] This therapy, especially in combination with laser ablative therapy, can provide local ablative control and has also been shown to cause significant clinical response in patients who were not surgical candidates.[39,40]

Argon Plasma Coagulation

Another type of local endoscopic therapy for advanced esophageal and gastric cancer is argon plasma coagulation. During argon plasma coagulation, a jet of ionized argon gas is passed through a probe within an endoscope. The argon gas is ignited within the probe, creating argon plasma. This argon plasma is applied locally to the surface of the tumor. Endoscopic debridement is subsequently performed. Repeat endoscopy is often performed 48 to 72 hours after the initial argon plasma therapy to assess tumor response, further debride tissue, or possible reapply therapy.[41] Retrospective reviews of argon plasma coagulation have shown that it may have some use in the control of local disease or in managing occluded stents, but it does not provide durable relief of dysphagia in the patient with an obstruction.[42]

Cryoablation

Endoscopic cryoablation is a local ablative therapy in which an endoscopist applies a spray of either liquid nitrogen or rapidly expanding carbon dioxide gas to the tumor tissue. The esophageal or gastric mucosa is exposed to the cryoablative spray for 10 to 20 seconds and then allowed to thaw. Multiple freeze/thaw cycles are repeated per session. Intracellular and extracellular ice crystals form during this process, and disrupt the integrity of the cancer cell membranes. This treatment causes immediate cytotoxicity and induces apoptosis in cancer cells. Sessions are generally repeated 6 to 8 weeks later.[43] Similar to the other local ablative therapies discussed, the results of cryoablative therapy are generally not durable in the relief of dysphagia, but can certainly be used in a multimodal approach to palliate dysphagia or obstruction in patients with advanced esophageal or gastric cancer (**Fig. 5**).[44,45]

Palliation of Dysphagia and Obstruction: Surgery

Esophageal cancer

Palliation of dysphagia in advanced esophageal cancer via esophagectomy or esophageal bypass procedures is generally saved as a last resort. Owing to the mortality and morbidity associated with such procedures in patients with a short life expectancy, surgery has fallen out of favor when compared with local endoscopic therapies to include dilation and stenting and other local ablative therapies.

Historically, before the advent of advanced endoscopic therapy, esophageal bypass was considered in the palliation of advanced esophageal cancer. Esophageal bypass has been described by a variety of surgeons via multiple techniques. The external drainage method,[46] the Postlethwait method,[47] the Kirschner method,[48] and ileocolonic bypass[49] are the most commonly described procedures. All of these procedures seek to exclude the existing esophagus with its advanced tumor and use a conduit (either gastric or terminal ileum and colon), which is anastomosed to the proximal esophagus to allow for resumption of oral intake. There is also some type of second anastomosis in all of these procedures to allow for drainage of the distal esophagus, except for the external drainage procedure, which uses an esophagostomy for drainage.[50] In some patients, the least morbid and simplest diversion is a loop cervical esophagostomy or "spit fistula" (**Fig. 6**).

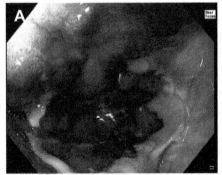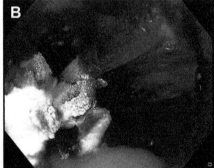

Fig. 5. Endoscopic cryotherapy of an esophageal tumor. In this patient, an upper endoscopy was performed and the area of tumor was identified. (*A*) An applicator was passed through the endoscope and the spray cryotherapy was applied to the endoluminal tumor. (*B*) After spray cryotherapy, the tumor demonstrates visible ice crystals.

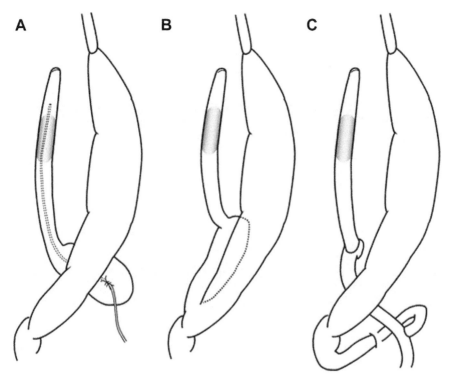

Fig. 6. Esophageal bypass via the (*A*) external drainage procedure, (*B*) Postlethwait method, and (*C*) the Kirschner method of esophageal bypass. (*From* Nakajima Y, Kawada K, Tokairin Y et al. Retrospective analyses of esophageal bypass surgery for patients with esophagorespiratory fistulas caused by esophageal carcinomas. World J Surg 2016;40:1158–64; with permission.)

Palliation of Dysphagia and Obstruction: Surgery

Gastric cancer

Similar to advanced esophageal cancer, endoluminal therapies are very popular and effective in the management of advanced gastric cancer with dysphagia or gastric outlet obstruction. Palliative surgery to relieve gastric outlet obstruction is still used in select patients and is more common as a palliative measure in the gastric cancer population than the esophageal cancer population. Surgery includes bypass procedures such as gastrojejunostomy as well as palliative resection.

Retrospective studies have shown that, in patients with gastric cancer and gastric outlet obstruction, endoscopic stenting when compared with surgery (both gastrojejunostomy and palliative resection) resulted in a faster improvement in oral intake, faster symptom relief, and shorter hospitalization. Complication rates, hospital readmissions, biliary obstruction, and receipt of chemotherapy were similar. The median symptom-free duration was longer in patients after gastrojejunostomy and palliative resection, and overall survival were longest in the palliative resection group.[22,24] These data are subject to selection bias, but suggest a potential benefit of surgical intervention in an appropriately selected patient population. Palliative resection even in stage IV disease may confer a survival advantage, but this type of resection is not the standard of care[4] and should generally only be considered in fit patients undergoing a palliative procedure for gastric outlet obstruction.

Bleeding

Another common complication of advanced gastric and esophageal cancer is bleeding. Patients may present with both lower volume intermittent bleeding from their tumor or brisk bleeding that affects hemodynamics if the tumor erodes into a nearby vessel. Herein we discuss treatment options for palliate bleeding in patients with advanced esophageal and gastric cancer.

Endoscopic therapy is the first-line treatment for palliation of bleeding in patients with esophageal and gastric cancer. Argon plasma coagulation, cryoablation, Nd:YAG laser therapy, and the application of endoscopic clips are the most commonly described methods.[40,42,51] If endoscopic therapies fail to control bleeding, other modalities such as radiation for diffuse tumor bleeding or tumor embolization for more brisk bleeding should be considered.

Perforation

Perforation is also a complication of advanced gastric and esophageal cancer. In small, contained perforations that are amenable to endoscopic stenting in the clinically stable patient, this is generally the preferred approach.[11,38] In patients with large perforations or patients who are critically ill, surgery is often required, assuming this is within the patient's goals of care. Regarding esophageal cancer, wide drainage, debridement, esophagostomy, jejunostomy, or some combination of these modalities is generally the preferred approach in these patients.[52]

Regarding perforated gastric cancer, surgical therapy may include an omental patch, wedge resection, or gastrectomy. A recent metaanalysis showed that, in cases of perforated gastric cancer where the surgeon was able to achieve an R0 resection at the time of operation for perforation, the overall survival was improved compared with those who did not receive an R0 resection.[53] Unfortunately, perforation is generally a feature of advanced tumors where an R0 resection may not be possible. The extent of the disease and the patient's fitness and comorbidities should be considered when operating for perforated gastric cancer.

Nutritional support

Given the location of both esophageal and gastric cancers within the alimentary tract, it is common for patients to experience difficulty obtaining adequate nutrition related to their obstructive symptoms. It is important to include a discussion of possible nutritional support and the inclusion of a registered dietician on the multidisciplinary team is of great importance. The discussion of possible nutritional support should include the current degree of dysphagia and ability of the patient to maintain oral intake, the life expectancy of the patient, the previous therapy undergone by the patient, and of course the patient's goals of care.

Nutritional support: Gastrostomy

Patients with esophageal or gastroesophageal junction cancer who do not have a history of significant prior abdominal surgery are likely good candidates for a percutaneous endoscopic gastrostomy feeding tubes. These tubes can even be placed in the setting of advanced tumors.

Nutritional support: Jejunostomy

Patients with gastric cancer or potentially resectable esophageal cancer requiring nutritional support generally undergo the placement of a jejunostomy feeding tube. This procedure can be performed open, laparoscopically, or even percutaneously by centers with advanced endoscopy.

Nutritional support: Parenteral nutrition

Parenteral nutrition in the setting of advanced esophageal or gastric cancer is generally limited to selected short-term cases. It is often reserved for those patients awaiting placement of an enteral delivery system or in those recovering from complications or surgery in very specific situations. Enteral feeding is highly preferred owing to potential infections, electrolyte abnormalities, liver abnormalities, and the cost associated with the use of parenteral nutrition.[54]

Life-Prolonging Therapy in Unresectable Esophageal or Gastric Cancer

Chemoradiotherapy for advanced unresectable esophageal cancer

Chemoradiotherapy is the standard therapy for unresectable esophageal cancer and should also be considered in the patient who is unfit for esophagectomy owing to medical reasons.[5] Studies from the Radiation Therapy Oncology Group (RTOG) 8501 showed that in patients with unresectable esophageal cancer randomized to either radiotherapy alone (64 Gy) or chemoradiotherapy (50 Gy and cisplatin), the median survival was 12.5 months in the chemoradiotherapy group and 8.9 months in the group who received radiotherapy alone ($P = .001$).[55,56] In the most recent update of this trial data, the 5-year overall survival was 26% in the chemoradiotherapy group compared with 0% in the radiotherapy alone group. Local recurrence and distant metastatic disease were also improved in the chemoradiotherapy group compared with the radiotherapy alone group.[55]

Given the advantage of chemotherapy shown by RTOG 850, studies have tried to elucidate the optimal chemotherapy regimen for definitive chemoradiation. Within the PRODIGE/ACCORD trial, patients with advanced esophageal or gastroesophageal junction cancer were randomized to either FOLFOX (leucovorin/5-fluoracil [5-FU]/oxaliplatin) or 5-FU and cisplatin in combination with radiation therapy.[57] There were no differences in the overall survival between the groups (3-year overall survival of 19.9% with FOLFOX vs 26.9% with cisplatin/5-FU). Additionally, response rates were not significantly different and there were no overall differences noted in the rates of toxicity.

Chemoradiotherapy for advanced unresectable gastric cancer

Chemoradiotherapy is also the standard of care for unresectable gastric cancer. As discussed, the RTOG 8501 trial, which included gastroesophageal junction tumors as well as solely esophageal tumors, demonstrated the benefit of the addition of chemotherapy to radiotherapy at improving survival for patients with unresectable cancer.[55,56] Chemotherapy regimens are also similar to those for esophageal cancer, as the PRODIGE/ACCORD trial results drive the use of both FOLFOX and 5-FU plus cisplatin regimens.

Also important in the treatment of advanced gastric cancer is the use of targeted therapy. HER2 was found to be overexpressed in 20% of gastric and gastroesophageal junction tumors[58] and thus its use as a target in gastric cancer therapy was investigated. The Trastuzumab for Gastric Cancer (ToGA) study was an open-label, international, phase 3, randomized, controlled trial that demonstrated that patients whose tumors overexpressed HER2 and who received chemotherapy (cisplatin plus capecitabine or cisplatin plus 5-FU) along with the targeted HER2 antibody trastuzumab had improved overall survival as compared with chemotherapy alone (13.8 months vs 11.1 months; $P = .0046$).[59] In addition to HER2, vascular endothelial growth factor–targeted therapies have been investigated in the treatment of gastric cancer, with mixed results.[60] Vascular endothelial growth factor receptor-2 has also been studied in populations with advanced gastric cancer and a targeted antibody against vascular endothelial growth factor receptor-2 is approved as a second-line agent.[61]

DISCUSSION

The palliative management of esophageal and gastric cancer should be approached in a multidisciplinary fashion, always holding the patient's goals of care at the center of the treatment discussion. For patients who wish to pursue aggressive treatment, chemoradiotherapy is the standard of care in both esophageal and gastric cancers. It is common for these patients to display significant symptomatology related to their disease, which can be addressed via multiple methods. Endoscopic treatments are now well-established as beneficial techniques to relieve dysphagia, obstruction, and bleeding. Surgery may also be warranted in certain situations, but a clear discussion with the patient about the goals of therapy and its associated risks is paramount. It is crucial to understand the patient's disease, the therapies available, and the patient's wishes when selecting the most appropriate treatment plan. Palliative therapy in advanced esophageal and gastric cancer seeks to balance the patient's desire to extend their life while simultaneously preserving a reasonable quality of life.

ACKNOWLEDGMENTS

The authors appreciate the endoscopic images provided by Sachin Wani, MD, and Hazzam Ahmad, MD, from the Department of Gastroenterology at the University of Colorado School of Medicine.

REFERENCES

1. National Cancer Institute; Surveillance E, and end results program. Cancer Stat Facts: Stomach Cancer. In. 2017.
2. National Cancer Institute; Surveillance, Epidemiology, and End Results program. Cancer Stat Facts: Esophageal Cancer. 2017.
3. Dunn GP. Surgical palliative care: recent trends and developments. Surg Clin North Am 2011;91:277–92, vii.
4. National Comprehensive Cancer Network. NCCN Clinical Practice Guidelines in Oncology Gastric Cancer. 2018; 2.2018.
5. National Comprehensive Cancer Network. NCCN clinical practice guidelines in Oncology esophageal and esophagogastric cancers. 2018; 2.2018.
6. Freeman RK, Ascioti AJ, Mahidhara RJ. Palliative therapy for patients with unresectable esophageal carcinoma. Surg Clin North Am 2012;92:1337–51.
7. Allum WH, Blazeby JM, Griffin SM, et al. Guidelines for the management of oesophageal and gastric cancer. Gut 2011;60:1449–72.
8. Knyrim K, Wagner HJ, Bethge N, et al. A controlled trial of an expansile metal stent for palliation of esophageal obstruction due to inoperable cancer. N Engl J Med 1993;329:1302–7.
9. Adler DG, Baron TH. Endoscopic palliation of malignant gastric outlet obstruction using self-expanding metal stents: experience in 36 patients. Am J Gastroenterol 2002;97:72–8.
10. Boyce HW Jr. Palliation of dysphagia of esophageal cancer by endoscopic lumen restoration techniques. Cancer Control 1999;6:73–83.
11. Kim JY, Kim SG, Lim JH, et al. Clinical outcomes of esophageal stents in patients with malignant esophageal obstruction according to palliative additional treatment. J Dig Dis 2015;16:575–84.
12. Sharma P, Kozarek R. Role of esophageal stents in benign and malignant diseases. Am J Gastroenterol 2010;105:258–73 [quiz: 274].

13. Pan YM, Pan J, Guo LK, et al. Covered versus uncovered self-expandable metallic stents for palliation of malignant gastric outlet obstruction: a systematic review and meta-analysis. BMC Gastroenterol 2014;14:170.

14. Acunas B, Rozanes I, Akpinar S, et al. Palliation of malignant esophageal strictures with self-expanding nitinol stents: drawbacks and complications. Radiology 1996;199:648–52.

15. Ell C, May A, Hahn EG. Gianturco-Z stents in the palliative treatment of malignant esophageal obstruction and esophagotracheal fistulas. Endoscopy 1995;27: 495–500.

16. Winkelbauer FW, Schofl R, Niederle B, et al. Palliative treatment of obstructing esophageal cancer with nitinol stents: value, safety, and long-term results. AJR Am J Roentgenol 1996;166:79–84.

17. Siersema PD, Schrauwen SL, van Blankenstein M, et al. Self-expanding metal stents for complicated and recurrent esophagogastric cancer. Gastrointest Endosc 2001;54:579–86.

18. Verschuur EM, Steyerberg EW, Kuipers EJ, et al. Effect of stent size on complications and recurrent dysphagia in patients with esophageal or gastric cardia cancer. Gastrointest Endosc 2007;65:592–601.

19. Raijman I, Siddique I, Ajani J, et al. Palliation of malignant dysphagia and fistulae with coated expandable metal stents: experience with 101 patients. Gastrointest Endosc 1998;48:172–9.

20. van Halsema EE, Rauws EA, Fockens P, et al. Self-expandable metal stents for malignant gastric outlet obstruction: a pooled analysis of prospective literature. World J Gastroenterol 2015;21:12468–81.

21. Endo S, Takiguchi S, Miyazaki Y, et al. Efficacy of endoscopic gastroduodenal stenting for gastric outlet obstruction due to unresectable advanced gastric cancer: a prospective multicenter study. J Surg Oncol 2014;109:208–12.

22. Keranen I, Kylanpaa L, Udd M, et al. Gastric outlet obstruction in gastric cancer: a comparison of three palliative methods. J Surg Oncol 2013;108:537–41.

23. Mansoor H, Zeb F. Enteral stents are safe and effective to relieve malignant gastric outlet obstruction in the elderly. J Gastrointest Cancer 2015;46:42–7.

24. Park JH, Song HY, Yun SC, et al. Gastroduodenal stent placement versus surgical gastrojejunostomy for the palliation of gastric outlet obstructions in patients with unresectable gastric cancer: a propensity score-matched analysis. Eur Radiol 2016;26:2436–45.

25. Lettmaier S, Strnad V. Intraluminal brachytherapy in oesophageal cancer: defining its role and introducing the technique. J Contemp Brachytherapy 2014;6:236–41.

26. Sur RK, Donde B, Levin VC, et al. Fractionated high dose rate intraluminal brachytherapy in palliation of advanced esophageal cancer. Int J Radiat Oncol Biol Phys 1998;40:447–53.

27. Taggar AS, Pitter KL, Cohen GN, et al. Endoluminal high-dose-rate brachytherapy for locally recurrent or persistent esophageal cancer. Brachytherapy 2018;17: 621–7.

28. Shishkova N, Kuznetsova O, Berezov T. Photodynamic therapy in gastroenterology. J Gastrointest Cancer 2013;44:251–9.

29. Yoon HY, Cheon YK, Choi HJ, et al. Role of photodynamic therapy in the palliation of obstructing esophageal cancer. Korean J Intern Med 2012;27:278–84.

30. Alexander GL, Wang KK, Ahlquist DA, et al. Does performance status influence the outcome of Nd:YAG laser therapy of proximal esophageal tumors? Gastrointest Endosc 1994;40:451–4.

31. Buset M, Dunham F, Baize M, et al. Nd-YAG laser, a new palliative alternative in the management of esophageal cancer. Endoscopy 1983;15:353–6.
32. Fleischer D. The Washington symposium on endoscopic laser therapy, April 18 and 19, 1985. Gastrointest Endosc 1985;31:397–400.
33. Maciel J, Barbosa J, Leal AS. Nd-YAG laser as a palliative treatment for malignant dysphagia. Eur J Surg Oncol 1996;22:69–73.
34. Naveau S, Chiesa A, Poynard T, et al. Endoscopic Nd-YAG laser therapy as palliative treatment for esophageal and cardial cancer. Parameters affecting long-term outcome. Dig Dis Sci 1990;35:294–301.
35. Renwick P, Whitton V, Moghissi K. Combined endoscopic laser therapy and brachytherapy for palliation of oesophageal carcinoma: a pilot study. Gut 1992; 33:435–8.
36. Moreira LS, Coelho RC, Sadala RU, et al. The use of ethanol injection under endoscopic control to palliate dysphagia caused by esophagogastric cancer. Endoscopy 1994;26:311–4.
37. Ramakrishnaiah VP, Ramkumar J, Pai D. Intratumoural injection of absolute alcohol in carcinoma of gastroesophageal junction for palliation of dysphagia. Ecancermedicalscience 2014;8:395.
38. Carazzone A, Bonavina L, Segalin A, et al. Endoscopic palliation of oesophageal cancer: results of a prospective comparison of Nd:YAG laser and ethanol injection. Eur J Surg 1999;165:351–6.
39. Robles-Jara C, Robles-Medranda C. Endoscopic chemotherapy with 5-fluorouracil in advanced gastric cancer. J Gastrointest Cancer 2010;41:75–8.
40. Wang Y, Zhou C, Jia J, et al. Endoscopic Nd:YAG laser therapy combined with local chemotherapy of superficial carcinomas of the oesophagus and gastric cardia. Lasers Med Sci 2001;16:299–303.
41. Wahab PJ, Mulder CJ, den Hartog G, et al. Argon plasma coagulation in flexible gastrointestinal endoscopy: pilot experiences. Endoscopy 1997;29:176–81.
42. Akhtar K, Byrne JP, Bancewicz J, et al. Argon beam plasma coagulation in the management of cancers of the esophagus and stomach. Surg Endosc 2000; 14:1127–30.
43. Vignesh S, Hoffe SE, Meredith KL, et al. Endoscopic therapy of neoplasia related to Barrett's esophagus and endoscopic palliation of esophageal cancer. Cancer Control 2013;20:117–29.
44. Goetz M, Malek NP, Kanz L, et al. Cryorecanalization for in-stent recanalization in the esophagus. Gastroenterology 2014;146:1168–70.
45. Greenwald BD, Dumot JA, Abrams JA, et al. Endoscopic spray cryotherapy for esophageal cancer: safety and efficacy. Gastrointest Endosc 2010;71:686–93.
46. Hihara J, Hamai Y, Emi M, et al. Esophageal bypass operation prior to definitive chemoradiotherapy in advanced esophageal cancer with tracheobronchial invasion. Ann Thorac Surg 2014;97:290–5.
47. Postlethwait R. Technique for isoperistaltic gastric tube for esophageal bypass. Ann Surg 1979;189:673.
48. Roeher HD, Horeyseck G. The Kirschner bypass operation—a palliation for complicated esophageal carcinoma. World J Surg 1981;5:543–6.
49. Kawano T, Nishikage T, Kawada K, et al. Subcutaneous reconstruction using ileocolon with preserved ileocolic vessels following esophagectomy or in esophageal bypass operation. Dig Surg 2009;26:200–4.
50. Nakajima Y, Kawada K, Tokairin Y, et al. Retrospective analyses of esophageal bypass surgery for patients with esophagorespiratory fistulas caused by esophageal carcinomas. World J Surg 2016;40:1158–64.

51. Shah MB, Schnoll-Sussman F. Novel use of cryotherapy to control bleeding in advanced esophageal cancer. Endoscopy 2010;42(Suppl 2):E46.
52. Nirula R. Esophageal perforation. Surg Clin North Am 2014;94:35–41.
53. Mahar AL, Brar SS, Coburn NG, et al. Surgical management of gastric perforation in the setting of gastric cancer. Gastric Cancer 2012;15(Suppl 1):S146–52.
54. Rivadeneira DE, Evoy D, Fahey TJ 3rd, et al. Nutritional support of the cancer patient. CA Cancer J Clin 1998;48:69–80.
55. Cooper JS, Guo MD, Herskovic A, et al. Chemoradiotherapy of locally advanced esophageal cancer: long-term follow-up of a prospective randomized trial (RTOG 85-01). Radiation Therapy Oncology Group. JAMA 1999;281:1623–7.
56. Herskovic A, Martz K, al-Sarraf M, et al. Combined chemotherapy and radiotherapy compared with radiotherapy alone in patients with cancer of the esophagus. N Engl J Med 1992;326:1593–8.
57. Conroy T, Galais MP, Raoul JL, et al. Definitive chemoradiotherapy with FOLFOX versus fluorouracil and cisplatin in patients with oesophageal cancer (PRODIGE5/ACCORD17): final results of a randomised, phase 2/3 trial. Lancet Oncol 2014;15:305–14.
58. Janjigian YY, Werner D, Pauligk C, et al. Prognosis of metastatic gastric and gastroesophageal junction cancer by HER2 status: a European and USA International collaborative analysis. Ann Oncol 2012;23:2656–62.
59. Bang YJ, Van Cutsem E, Feyereislova A, et al. Trastuzumab in combination with chemotherapy versus chemotherapy alone for treatment of HER2-positive advanced gastric or gastro-oesophageal junction cancer (ToGA): a phase 3, open-label, randomised controlled trial. Lancet 2010;376:687–97.
60. Ohtsu A, Shah MA, Van Cutsem E, et al. Bevacizumab in combination with chemotherapy as first-line therapy in advanced gastric cancer: a randomized, double-blind, placebo-controlled phase III study. J Clin Oncol 2011;29:3968–76.
61. Fuchs CS, Tomasek J, Yong CJ, et al. Ramucirumab monotherapy for previously treated advanced gastric or gastro-oesophageal junction adenocarcinoma (REGARD): an international, randomised, multicentre, placebo-controlled, phase 3 trial. Lancet 2014;383:31–9.

Moving?

Make sure your subscription moves with you!

To notify us of your new address, find your **Clinics Account Number** (located on your mailing label above your name), and contact customer service at:

Email: journalscustomerservice-usa@elsevier.com

800-654-2452 (subscribers in the U.S. & Canada)
314-447-8871 (subscribers outside of the U.S. & Canada)

Fax number: 314-447-8029

Elsevier Health Sciences Division
Subscription Customer Service
3251 Riverport Lane
Maryland Heights, MO 63043

*To ensure uninterrupted delivery of your subscription, please notify us at least 4 weeks in advance of move.

Printed and bound by CPI Group (UK) Ltd, Croydon, CR0 4YY

03/10/2024

01040407-0015